EMDR Therapy for CLINICIAN SELF-CARE

Marilyn Luber, PhD, is a licensed clinical psychologist in general private practice in Center City, Philadelphia, Pennsylvania. She was trained in eye movement desensitization and reprocessing (EMDR) in 1992 by Dr. Francine Shapiro, and now assists in EMDR Institute trainings as a facilitator and logistics coordinator. She has coordinated trainings in EMDR-related fields in the greater Philadelphia area since 1997. She teaches Facilitator and Supervisory trainings and other EMDR-related subjects both nationally and internationally, and was on the EMDR Task Force for Dissociative Disorders. She was on the founding board of directors of the EMDR International Association (EMDRIA) and served as the chair of the International Committee until June 1999. Currently, she is a facilitator in the EMDR Global Alliance, a group consisting of the leaders of all the EMDR associations who are working to support standards in EMDR worldwide. In 1997, Dr. Luber was given a Humanitarian Services Award by the EMDR Humanitarian Association, and later, in 2003, she was presented with the EMDR International Association's award for "outstanding contribution and service to EMDRIA." In 2005, she was awarded the Francine Shapiro Award for "outstanding contribution and service to EMDR." In 2009, she edited *Eye Movement Desensitization and Reprocessing (EMDR) Scripted Protocols: Basics and Special Situations* and *Eye Movement Desensitization and Reprocessing (EMDR) Scripted Protocols: Special Populations* published by Springer Publishing Company. Several years later, in 2012, she edited Springer's first CD-ROM books, *Eye Movement Desensitization and Reprocessing (EMDR) Scripted Protocols With Summary Sheets CD-ROM Version: Basics and Special Situations* and *Eye Movement Desensitization and Reprocessing (EMDR) Scripted Protocols With Summary Sheets CD-ROM Version: Special Populations*. In 2001, through EMDR-HAP (Humanitarian Assistance Programs), she published *Handbook for EMDR Clients* and it has been translated into eight languages. She has written the "Around the World" and "In the Spotlight" articles for the EMDRIA Newsletter four times a year since 1997. She has worked as a primary consultant for the FBI field division in Philadelphia. Dr. Luber has a general psychology practice, working with adolescents, adults, and couples, especially with complex posttraumatic stress disorder (C-PTSD), trauma and related issues, and dissociative disorders. She runs consultation groups for EMDR practitioners.

EMDR Therapy for CLINICIAN SELF-CARE

Edited by

Marilyn Luber, PhD

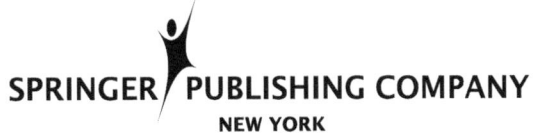

SPRINGER PUBLISHING COMPANY

NEW YORK

Copyright © 2015 Springer Publishing Company, LLC

All rights reserved.

No part of this publication may be reproduced, stored in a retrieval system, or transmitted in any form or by any means, electronic, mechanical, photocopying, recording, or otherwise, without the prior permission of Springer Publishing Company, LLC, or authorization through payment of the appropriate fees to the Copyright Clearance Center, Inc., 222 Rosewood Drive, Danvers, MA 01923, 978-750-8400, fax 978-646-8600, info@copyright.com or on the Web at www.copyright.com.

Springer Publishing Company, LLC
11 West 42nd Street
New York, NY 10036
www.springerpub.com

Acquisitions Editor: Sheri W. Sussman
Composition: S4Carlisle

ISBN: 978-0-8261-3339-7
e-book ISBN: 978-0-8261-3224-6

Content herein is excerpted from *Implementing EMDR Early Mental Health Interventions for Man-Made and Natural Disasters: Models, Scripted Protocols, and Summary Sheets*, edited by Marilyn Luber. © Springer Publishing Company, LLC. The Foreword, Preface, Acknowledgments, and section introductions have been included herein in their entirety.

The author and the publisher of this Work have made every effort to use sources believed to be reliable to provide information that is accurate and compatible with the standards generally accepted at the time of publication. The author and publisher shall not be liable for any special, consequential, or exemplary damages resulting, in whole or in part, from the readers' use of, or reliance on, the information contained in this book. The publisher has no responsibility for the persistence or accuracy of URLs for external or third-party Internet websites referred to in this publication and does not guarantee that any content on such websites is, or will remain, accurate or appropriate.

Implementing EMDR early mental health interventions for man-made and natural disasters : models, scripted protocols, and summary sheets/edited by Marilyn Luber.
  p. ; cm.
Implementing eye movement desensitization reprocessing early mental health interventions for man-made and natural disasters
  Includes bibliographical references and index.
  ISBN-13: 978-0-8261-9921-8
  ISBN-10: 0-8261-9921-6
  ISBN-13: 978-0-8261-3224-6 (e-book)
  ISBN-13: 978-0-8261-2957-4 (CD-ROM)
    I. Luber, Marilyn, editor of compilation. II. Title: Implementing eye movement desensitization reprocessing early mental health interventions for man-made and natural disasters.
  [DNLM: 1. Stress Disorders, Traumatic--therapy.   2. Cross-Cultural Comparison.   3. Disasters.   4. Eye Movement Desensitization Reprocessing. WM 172.5]
  RC552.T7
  616.85'21—dc23
                                                                                           2013021409

Special discounts on bulk quantities of our books are available to corporations, professional associations, pharmaceutical companies, health care organizations, and other qualifying groups.

If you are interested in a custom book, including chapters from more than one of our titles, we can provide that service as well.

For details, please contact:
Special Sales Department, Springer Publishing Company, LLC
11 West 42nd Street, 15th Floor, New York, NY 10036-8002
Phone: 877-687-7476 or 212-431-4370; Fax: 212-941-7842
E-mail: sales@springerpub.com

Printed in the United States of America.

To my mother, who has been going through her own recent trauma
with the spirit and true determination
that she has always displayed throughout her life:
a role model for us all.

Epigraph

We are all responsible for the world we live in. Worldwide, clinicians are forging bonds that transcend countries and ideologies. Bonds that can help heal the trauma and pain that lead to ongoing violence and suffering. To make a difference that effects generations to come—don't leave it to anyone else. We all have to take a part in it.

—Francine Shapiro

Contents

Contributors xi

Foreword xiii
Robert Gelbach

Preface xv

Acknowledgments xxix

PART I
EMDR and Clinician Self-Care: Recent Trauma Response

Chapter 1   Self-Care for EMDR Practitioners 5
Neal Daniels

Summary Sheet: Self-Care for EMDR Practitioners 7
Marilyn Luber

Chapter 2   Community Trauma: A Blueprint for Support and Treatment for Trauma Recovery Network (TRN) Responders From the Newtown, CT, Tragedy 9
Karen Alter-Reid

Summary Sheet: Community Trauma: A Blueprint for Support and Treatment for Trauma Recovery Network (TRN) Responders From the Newtown, CT, Tragedy 17
Marilyn Luber

Chapter 3   Vicarious Trauma and EMDR 21
Derek Farrell

Summary Sheet: Vicarious Trauma and EMDR 39
Marilyn Luber

Chapter 4   Worst Case Scenarios in Recent Trauma Response 47
Ignacio Jarero and Susana Uribe

Summary Sheet: Worst Case Scenarios in Recent Trauma Response 53
Marilyn Luber

Appendix A: Worksheets 57

Appendix B: EMDR Worldwide Associations and Other Resources 76

References and Bibliography 83

Contributors

Karen Alter-Reid, PhD, is a clinical psychologist specializing in the treatment of traumatic stress. She integrates EMDR, relational psychotherapy, sensorimotor psychotherapy, hypnosis, and HeartMath into her work with clients. She worked on several Humanitarian Assistance Program projects in New Orleans following Hurricanes Katrina and Rita. This included providing treatment to first responders, EMDR clinicians, and locals and providing EMDR specialty training and consultation. She presented the research project *Therapy for Therapists: Impact of Intensive EMDR Treatment Post-Katrina* at the EMDRIA 2011 conference. Dr. Alter-Reid is co-coordinator of the Fairfield County Trauma Recovery Network in CT and, along with HAP, is actively involved in the aftermath of the Newtown/Sandy Hook tragedy, where she treats first responders, organizes trainings, and cares for the local EMDR clinicians. She is an EMDR-HAP Trainer, and EMDRIA Specialty Presenter, and Southwestern CT EMDRIA Regional co-coordinator.

Neal Daniels, PhD, received his MA in Social Psychology from the New School for Social Research and his PhD from Kansas University and Menninger Clinic. In 1981, he left his long service as a Family Therapist with the Philadelphia Child Guidance Clinic to become Director of the newly formed program for PTSD at the Philadelphia VA Hospital where EMDR became an integral part of the treatment program. His article, "Post-Traumatic Stress Disorder and Competence to Stand Trial," was published in the *Journal of Psychiatry and Law*, Spring 1984. His research on the EMDR treatment of triggers remains unfinished due to his retirement and final illness.

Derek Farrell, PhD, is a senior lecturer in psychology at the University of Worcester, honorary senior lecturer at University of Birmingham, EMDR-Europe accredited trainer and consultant, chartered psychologist with the British Psychological Society, and an Accredited CBT Psychotherapist with the British Association of Behavioural and Cognitive Psychotherapies (BABCP). He is president of EMDR-Europe Humanitarian Assistance Programmes, is a member of the EMDR-Europe Science and Research Committee, co-chair of EMDR-Europe Practice Sub-Committee and is a member of the EMDR-Europe Board, past president of EMDR UK and Ireland, and Past Chair EMDR UK and Ireland Accreditation Committee. He has been involved in a number of Humanitarian Assistance programs training mental health workers in the aftermath of the Turkish and Pakistan earthquakes and the Indian Ocean tsunami. Dr. Farrell is presently involved in a long-term project in Pakistan developing mental health psychological trauma services mainly around the intervention of EMDR. In 1995, he commenced a PhD in Psychology researching survivor's experiences of sexual abuse perpetrated by clergy and as a consequence has written several publications on this subject matter. He completed his doctoral studies in 2003. In October 2012, he moved to the University of Worcester, being involved with both undergraduate and postgraduate programs. In addition he is an honorary EMDR consultant/cognitive behavioral psychotherapist with Birmingham and Solihull Mental Health NHS Trust. He has had over 25 articles published in academic journals and written two book chapters. Dr. Farrell is actively engaged in EMDR research and supervision of PhD studies relating to EMDR.

Ignacio Jarero, PhD, EdD, MT, is a trainer of trainers, EMDRIA and EMDR-Ibero-America cofounder, and approved consultant. He is cofounder and president of EMDR-Mexico, AMAMECRISIS, and International Center of Psychotraumatology. In 2007, he received the EMDR-Ibero-America Francine Shapiro Award and, in 2008, the Argentinian Society of Psychotrauma (ISTSS Affiliate) awarded him the Psychotrauma Trajectory Award. He is a trainer for the International Critical Incident Stress Foundation and Green Cross Academy of Traumatology. Dr. Jarero is coauthor of the EMDR Integrative Group Treatment Protocol that has been applied successfully with disaster survivors worldwide. He has presented workshops and has published articles on EMDR, crisis intervention, and compassion fatigue. Since 1997, he has been involved in humanitarian projects in Latin America and Europe.

Susana G. Uribe Ramirez, MA, is the vice president of EMDR-Mexico, an EMDR Institute facilitator, and an EMDR Ibero-America–approved consultant. In addition, she is a clinical psychotraumatologist for Green Cross Academy of Traumatology. She specializes in treating adult victims of trauma and complicated grief. She is a consultant in trauma, loss, and mourning processes, and an international lecturer on utilizing EMDR with trauma, loss, and grief.

Foreword

Foreword taken from *Implementing EMDR Early Mental Health Interventions for Man-Made and Natural Disasters: Models, Scripted Protocols, and Summary Sheets*, edited by Marilyn Luber. © Springer Publishing Company, LLC.

Human beings are born into the care and company of others. From our first breath, our lives are a progressive encounter and mastery of environing stresses, mediated to an overwhelming degree by the web of social relationships and cultural meanings that sustain us throughout our lives. Sometimes, our individual capacity to manage excessive stress derails us and we may need assistance to reestablish a healthy coping capability. The evolution of mental health resources in developed countries has expanded the availability and efficacy of such assistance for individuals overcome by personal traumatic stress in normal times.

But disaster is not "normal"; in fact it is a severe disruption of the normal context in which we can find our bearings and rely on familiar systems of support. Disaster brings very high levels of traumatic stress at the same time that it undermines the usual coping resources and systems of care that may mitigate trauma or support healing.

The authors collected in this volume have been creative participants in the first generation of therapists who employed EMDR as a clinical treatment for posttraumatic stress disorder and related conditions. They know firsthand what research has confirmed—that EMDR is an effective and efficacious treatment for trauma in both children and adults, across all cultures and groups where it has been employed. It was only natural that they would want to apply this therapy to the massive trauma issues arising in modern day disasters, whether these arise from natural events (earthquake, tsunami, hurricane) or man-made disasters (warfare, flight from persecution, or famine).

However, although much psychotherapy has advanced in the past century in some parts of the world, it remains substantially underdeveloped where most of the world's people live. Moreover, even in places where psychotherapy is well-established it is not widely available at all socioeconomic levels. And most important, it is not widely understood by those who coordinate disaster response nationally or internationally that psychotherapy has a valuable role in early disaster intervention.

Clinician volunteers from the EMDR Humanitarian Assistance Program (HAP) and sister organizations have not been discouraged by these circumstances. As the following chapters recount, they have rolled up their sleeves and entered into the scene of disaster determined to find out how principles of EMDR can be best utilized to reduce trauma and increase the coping capacity of disaster survivors so that the goals of recovery and adaptation can be more fully and rapidly attained.

I had the privilege of meeting and working with many of the authors collected here while I served as Executive Director of HAP. They accomplished much by their direct service to survivors and by their teaching of useful skills to local caregivers. But they also learned much about the capacity of other cultures to support the coping efforts of their members, about the need for mental health response to blend collaboratively into the overall efforts of disaster responders to also address medical, nutritional, shelter, security, economic, and other needs. They learned the importance of adapting the mental health response to the particular phase of disaster recovery, and to the need for special attention to the first responders and local human service workers confronting vicarious traumatization.

Surely one of the most universal lessons learned was that populations and public officials everywhere were rarely equipped in advance to grapple with the emergent mental health issues that arise out of a community-wide disaster. From this recognition has come a growing effort to develop in all countries a more widespread understanding of traumatic stress and its treatment. Especially because disasters tend to occur in those countries and populations that are least resilient, the efforts to build up public understanding of trauma and caregiver skills for stress reduction *before disaster strikes* seem most likely to mitigate the psychological toll of future disasters. That is why HAP has been particularly interested in developing Trauma Recovery Networks in all countries where HAP works.

In this latest insightful volume gathered and edited by Marilyn Luber, the authors have combined the lessons learned with personal accounts of how they proceeded. There is still much to be done to integrate mental health care effectively into disaster response worldwide, but this volume will help to point the way to best practices.

Robert Gelbach, PhD
Past Executive Director at EMDR Humanitarian Assistance Programs

Preface

Preface taken from *Implementing EMDR Early Mental Health Interventions for Man-Made and Natural Disasters: Models, Scripted Protocols, and Summary Sheets*, edited by Marilyn Luber. © Springer Publishing Company, LLC.

All of us familiar with EMDR have heard about Francine Shapiro's 1987 walk in the park and how she observed her own disturbing thoughts disappear. On reflection, she realized that her eye movements seemed to be resulting in a decrease of her once distressing thoughts. She was surprised and intrigued and tried it again with other thoughts. It worked again. She decided to try it with friends and when it worked again, she tried it with clients. She took this eye movement phenomenon and crafted a protocol based on the following elements:

- Incident: "Describe the memory from which you wish relief in terms of who was involved and what had happened."
- Picture: "Isolate a single picture that represents the entire memory (preferably the most traumatic point of the incident) and indicate who and what is in the picture."
- Negative cognition (NC): "What words about yourself or the incident best go with the picture?"
- SUD scale: "Imagine the traumatic scene and the words of the belief statement ___ (state the negative cognition) and assign a SUDs (subjective units of disturbance scale) where 0 = (neutral or calm) to 10 = (the worst you can think of), how does it feel?"
- Positive cognition (PC): "How would you like to feel instead?"
- Validity of cognition (VoC) for PC: On a 1 to 7 scale where 1 feels completely false and 7 feels completely true, how true does the new statement feel to you?" (Shapiro, 1989)

She called it Eye Movement Desensitization (EMD). Over time, as she observed the processing of many traumatic incidents by many clients, she believed that the results went beyond a desensitization effect and actually reprocessed and changed clients' perceptions of their traumas; she added an "R" for "Reprocessing" and renamed EMD to EMDR (Shapiro, 1991).

In 1989, the San Francisco Bay Area earthquake not only disrupted this community, it changed the way Francine viewed trauma that had recently/just occurred. As more and more clients came to her office to process their experiences of the quake, she noticed that something was different when she used her normal protocol for EMDR: It was not generalizing. Instead of targeting the memory and having the process link to the other associations related to the traumatic memory network, she had to be more actively engaged in helping clients target the next part of their earthquake experience. It was as if the parts were not yet integrated into a whole. She realized that the memories her clients were telling her had not yet consolidated and that she needed to figure out how to help them link into the memory networks associated with the event. The premise of EMDR is the Adaptive Information Processing Model (AIP; for more in-depth descriptions, see Shapiro, 1995, 2001, 2006; Shapiro, Kaslow, & Maxfield, 2007); this means that everyone has an inborn predisposition to move toward health and the internal ability to accomplish it. When this movement is obstructed (and not related to a lack of information or organic issues), it is probable that the experiences become dysfunctionally stored and unable to connect with other adaptive information. As a result, clients may have maladaptive images, perceptual distortions, emotions, and sensations that are "stuck" in trauma time, unable to process. That is, adaptive information is unable to link into the memory networks holding the dysfunctionally stored information. The goal becomes to enable the more adaptive information held in other neural networks to link into these dysfunctionally stored memories and facilitate normal memory processing.

In response to her clients' needs, she created the Protocol for Recent Traumatic Events (Shapiro, 1995; 2001). The protocol she crafted addressed how to reprocess the elements of an unconsolidated memory with little/no linkages. She started by obtaining a "narrative history" of the event. She wisely took each of the separate aspects of the memory her clients reported and treated each one of them as a separate target with the EMDR Standard procedure up to the installation of the positive cognition (PC). She thoughtfully decided to not go beyond that because clients would then have to pay attention to body sensations that would continue to be there, she reasoned, because the whole memory had yet to be completed. If there was a most disturbing element of the memory, she started there, if not, she followed clients' chronologies of the event. After the first part of the memory was completed, she did the others in chronological order.

To check the work, she asked clients to visualize the entire sequence of the event with their eyes closed as she figured they would be better able to concentrate on their experiences and associate to it. If they did notice that there was some residual distress, she asked them to stop and then she used the EMDR Procedure including the NC and PC. She had clients continue this process and repeat it—if needed—until the whole event could be experienced with no emotional, cognitive, or somatic change. By asking clients next to open their eyes and think of the whole event from start to finish, she could observe if they could also keep one foot in the present and one in the not-so-distant past. Then, she installed the PC. After this was done, she was ready to check and see if clients had any residual distress in their bodies that needed processing, so she had them do the body scan. When all of the different elements of the event were completed and the body scan was clear, she asked for any present stimuli such as triggers that resulted in a startle response, nightmares, or other reminders of the event that were still disturbing and she processed each trigger with her clients. Although she did not write about the future template in this section of her book, she discusses the 3-Pronged Protocol throughout it and so it is assumed that she includes this as well. Out of the devastating San Francisco Bay Area earthquake of 1989 came a new treatment for recent trauma.

Over the years, recognition of EMDR as a treatment has grown. In fact the following organizations are incorporating EMDR into their treatment guidelines: Clinical Division of the American Psychological Association (Chambless et al., 1998); United Kingdom Department of Health (2001); National Council for Mental Health (Israel) (Bleich, Kotler, Kutz, & Shalev, 2002); Clinical Resource Efficiency Support Team of the Northern Ireland Department of Health, Social Services and Public Safety, Belfast (CREST, 2003); Dutch National Steering Committee Guidelines Mental Health Care (2003); Stockholm: Medical Program Committee/Stockholm City Council, Sweden (Sjöblom et al., 2003); American Psychiatric Association (2004); Department of Veterans Affairs & Department of Defense (2004); French National Institute of Health and Medical Research (INSERM, 2004); Therapy Advisor (2004–2007); National Collaborating Center for Mental Health (2005); Australian Centre for Posttraumatic Mental Health (2007); Practice Guidelines of the International Society for Traumatic Stress Studies (Foa, 2009); California Evidence-Based Clearinghouse for Child Welfare (2010); and the Substance Abuse and Mental Health Services Administration (SAMHSA) National Registry of Evidence-Based Programs and Practices (SAMHSA, 2011) (retrieved from the EMDR Institute website [www.emdr.com] and Schubert & Lee [2009]). Only two of these guidelines include specific references to the use of EMDR with clients diagnosed with acute stress disorder (APA, 2004; Australian Centre for Posttraumatic Mental Health, 2007). The other guidelines designate EMDR as an evidence-based treatment for PTSD; however, it seems that all of the guidelines are referring to EMDR related to chronic PTSD (after 3 months).

Kutz, Resnick, and Dekel (2008) point out that information on "the biology and psychology of acute stress syndromes is relatively sparse," and they go on to suggest, based on their clinical experience with terror and accident victims, that the current idea of time-related definitions of acute, posttraumatic stress might need to be modified and gave the following example: "the border (4 weeks) between ASD and acute PTSD seems utterly arbitrary, and both ASD and acute PTSD seem to form a continuous acute stress (AS) Syndrome." In a similar vein, Mark Russell, Tammera Cooke, and Susan Rogers in their chapter, "EMDR and Effective Management of Acute Stress Injuries: Early Mental Health Intervention From a Military Perspective" ask a similar question, "What is the difference between 3 weeks and 6 days (acute stress disorder) and 4 weeks and a day (PTSD)?" They note that after 4 weeks, the ASD diagnosis automatically converts to PTSD and EMDR is one of the few "A-level" trauma-targeted psychotherapies for PTSD. Also, they cite clinical case studies reported by Russell (2006) and Wesson and Gould (2009) showing that EMDR treatment is successful when treating combat-related ASR and ASD for those on active duty in the military. They believe that this distinction is arbitrary and empirically unsupported.

Elan Shapiro (2012, p. 244), in his article looking at the field of early psychological intervention (EPI) after trauma and the place of EMDR, reports, "the state of current evidence about early response to trauma and subsequent disorders reveals a complex picture. Bryant, Creamer, O'Donnell, Silove, and McFarlane (2011), summarizing the findings of an ambitious study which investigated the extent to which ASD at 1 month predicts posttraumatic psychiatric disorders at 12 months after trauma, in a large sample from five Australian hospitals concluded that the ASD diagnosis has limited utility in identifying recent trauma-exposed individuals who are at high risk for PTSD . . . however . . . most people diagnosed with ASD will suffer some psychiatric disorder a year later. . . . In contrast the overall utility of the diagnosis as an early screening strategy . . . is very limited because the majority of people who develop a disorder will not initially display full or subsyndromal ASD" (Bryant et al., 2011, p. 5).

Shapiro (2012, p. 244) discusses practical and ethical questions concerning the importance of treatment of ASD since so many go on to develop PTSD or other psychiatric disorders (Bryant, Friedman, Spiegel, Ursano, & Strain, 2010; Roberts, Kitchiner, Kenardy, & Bisson, 2009;) and the fact that PTSD is only one of several disorders that can result from trauma may mean that we could be overlooking an important group who go on to develop these disorders. Shapiro goes on to report (2012, p. 244), "The possibility of delayed-onset PTSD should also be remembered, as it was found to occur in up to 68% of cases, depending on definitions (Andrews, Brewin, Philpott, & Stewart, 2007)." Other concerns, also in Shapiro's article (2012, p. 242), are mentioned by Vanitallie (2002), such as "the dysregulation of the metabolic system, stemming from chronic stress, and attempts to accommodate it (allostatic load) contributes to the development of a variety of illnesses, as well as certain disorders of immune function" or McFarlane (2010a, 2010b) who states, "The association with cardiovascular risk factors and inflammatory markers indicates that exposure to traumatic stress leads to a general disruption of an individual's underlying homeostasis" (2010b, p. 5). The high cost to individuals and to society is evident.

Although there are a number of PTSD studies concerning the efficacy of EMDR, there are very few reports on the effect of EMDR on AS; undoubtedly, more research would be helpful in more clearly defining these diagnoses and the best interventions for them. The Cochrane review of psychological interventions looked at psychological interventions within the first 3 months after a traumatic event, and was unable to recommend any early psychological intervention for general immediate use after a critical incident (Roberts, Kitchiner, Kenardy, & Bisson, 2008, 2009). However, EMDR-based protocols are being used with increasing frequency in individual or group formats to address the traumatic symptoms subsequent to man-made and natural disasters and from the reports and the research that is beginning to be published, survivors' traumatic symptoms are decreasing.

In this text, there are several different protocols used to address AS. Francine's original EMD Protocol was brought back into circulation in the *Military and Post-Disaster Response Manual* (Shapiro, 2004) for emergency situations such as in frontline military operations. In EMD, the client is returned to the target frequently, the SUD level is checked, and the focus is on the target without moving down the associative tracks to other events/situations. This is a highly structured intervention meant to keep the client focused in emergency situations. Emergency room treatments have also been utilized as in Gary Quinn's Emergency Response Procedure (ERP) for stabilization and Judith Guedalia and Frances Yoeli's EMDR Emergency Room and Wards Protocol (EMDR-ER©) to help get patients who had been traumatized functioning again and able to leave the ER. Kutz, Resnick, and Dekel (2008) used a "modified, abridged, single session" EMDR protocol for AS syndromes using mainly the BLS element of the Standard EMDR Protocol without the cognitive processing elements while focusing on the most distressing sensory, bodily experience, or cognitive preoccupation related to the traumatic incident and rated with the SUDs. Sets are continued until there is a decrease in distress. Their results showed that with this intervention 50% had complete relief and 27% experienced substantial relief of their acutely stressed patients and concluded that this brief variation can be useful for victims of large scale disaster as well as trauma victims in hospitals and outpatient situations. Russell has used EMD; he targets only a single memory with the image, NC, emotions, SUDs, and location of body sensation with BLS to assist with crisis intervention and reduce the primary symptoms associated with the precipitating event without following free associations that are unrelated to the target. He uses a modified EMDR (Mod-EMDR) script that he has adapted from the EMD script; here, the target can be a single incident target memory or a representative worst memory from a group of memories related to the specific event. Russell reports using these scripts with patients after a near or immediate aftermath of exposure to a severe or potentially traumatic event or when patients present with severe acute stress responses or combat and operational stress reactions.

Elan Shapiro and Brurit Laub (2008) created a comprehensive protocol called "Recent Traumatic Episode Protocol" (R-TEP) that expands the existing protocols of EMD, ER-related protocols, and EMDR together and includes ways to contain and keep clients safe while processing. Their protocol introduces four important concepts: the Traumatic Episode, the Episode Narrative, the Google Search, and Telescopic Processing.

R-TEP was used and research done with victims of a terrorist bombing in Gungoren, Istanbul (Altan Aytun et al., 2010). The participants were children and adults who scored high on the IES and the PTSD Symptom Checklist. R-TEP (incorporating EMD and Recent Event Protocols) was used with the adult participants who were seen weekly to work only on the trauma of the bombing; participants completed an IES prior to each session. The number of sessions was restricted to the completion of EMD and R-TEP. The data analyses demonstrate that EMDR was effective with the adults and helped in the prevention of PTSD and recommended the use of EMDR as a crises intervention tool. The positive effect was maintained at a 3-month follow up. Tofani and Wheeler (2012) applied R-TEP in three different cases, observing markers such as distance concerning the trauma, a decrease in negative affect, access to information that is more adaptive, and changes in measures such as the SUDs, the VoC scale, and the revised IES-R, indicating changes in the perception of the traumatic memory. All three clients reported therapeutic changes in behavior and functioning. The EMDR R-TEP was used with over 2,000 survivors of recent earthquakes in northern Italy with pre- and posttreatment data collected showing changes in posttraumatic stress (Shapiro & Fernandez, 2013). Also, it was used with survivors from the recent earthquake in eastern Turkey in 2012 (Shapiro, 2012, p. 244).

Ignacio Jarero and Lucina Artigas created a different modification of Shapiro's (2001) Protocol for Recent Traumatic Events provided in an individual treatment format to clients suffering from recent ongoing trauma called the "EMDR Protocol for Recent Critical Incidents" (EMDR-PRECI). It was developed in the field under extremely dangerous circumstances to treat critical incidents where related stressful events continued for an extended time (often more than 6 months) and where there was no posttrauma period of safety for memory consolidation. Two randomized controlled trials (RCT) with the EMDR-PRECI have been published with delayed treatment designs supporting the efficacy of EMDR-PRECI in reducing symptoms after a 7.2 earthquake in North Baja California, Mexico (Jarero, Artigas, & Luber, 2011), and working with traumatized first responders responding to a human massacre situation (Jarero & Uribe, 2011, 2012).

An EMDR group protocol, the EMDR Integrative Group Treatment Protocol, was created in 1997 in Mexico after Hurricane Pauline (Artigas et al., 2000, 2009). Originally, this work was designed for children and combined the Standard EMDR Protocol with a group therapy model (Artigas et al., 2000; Jarero et al., 1999). However, it has been used with good success with disaster survivors from 7 years of age upward. There are a number of reports of its success worldwide (Aduriz, Knopfler, & Bluthgen, 2009; Errebo, Knipe, Forte, Karlin, & Altayli, 2008; Jarero et al., 2006, 2008), or with adaptations to meet the circumstances (Fernandez et al., 2004; Gelbach & Davis, 2007; Korkmazlar-Oral & Pamuk, 2002; Wilson, Tinker, Hofmann, Becker, & Marshall, 2000; Zaghrout-Hodali, Alissa, & Dodgson, 2008). Jarero and Artigas (2010) applied the EMDR-IGTP during 3 consecutive days to 20 adults in a Central American country with an ongoing geopolitical crisis. Results of this uncontrolled study showed decreases in scores on the SUDs and IES. Changes in the IES were maintained at a 14-week follow up even with ongoing crisis. Louise Maxfield (2008, p. 75) wrote that, "EMDR-IGTP has been found effective in several field trials and has been used for thousands of disaster survivors around the world."

The Imma Protocol (2009) was adapted from the IGTP and includes the Four Elements for Stress Management and group dynamic principles. Also, the Indian response team in Gujarat created an EMDR group protocol including the Butterfly Hug that was used with approximately 16,000 children in the area with positive results and decrease in traumatic symptoms.

There have been some cases described in the literature that discuss successful treatment of adults using EMD with two women, 1 month after the Great Hanshin-Awaji earthquake. They had been diagnosed with ASD. With both women, the SUDs decreased to 0 and the changes were maintained at a 5-month follow up (Ichii & Kumano, 1996).

Francine Shapiro's Protocol for Recent Traumatic Events was used with 9/11 survivors (Silver, Rogers, Knipe, & Colelli, 2005). They found that EMDR was a useful treatment intervention in the immediate aftermath of the event and later as well. In 2008, Colelli and Patterson found that their three cases demonstrated the usefulness of EMDR as a postdisaster treatment. It was only used in one case less than 3 months after 9/11; however, it was also found effective after 9 and 12 months. Fernandez (2002) used an average of 6.5 EMDR sessions for successful treatment with child survivors of the Molise earthquake in Italy; this was done over treatment cycles of 1 month, 3 months, and 1 year post incident. In 2008, Fernandez worked with a tsunami survivor diagnosed with acute PTSD and in a case study reported that after three EMDR sessions, the survivor was symptom free. The different forms of the EMDR protocol are being used quite actively in the EMDR community to relieve the distress of patients post disaster as has been illustrated above. Given the amount of catastrophes that we seem to be facing in the world on a more and more regular basis, it is an appropriate time for a book such as *Implementing EMDR Early Mental Health Interventions for Man-Made and Natural Disasters: Models, Scripted Protocols, and Summary Sheets*.

The seed for *Implementing EMDR Early Mental Health Interventions for Man-Made and Natural Disasters: Models, Scripted Protocols, and Summary Sheets* grew out of this author's many exposures to recent trauma over the years growing up: under the constant threat of nuclear holocaust; living through the Vietnam era; hearing about sexual assault from my clients and about motor vehicle accidents; learning EMDR in 1992 and how to treat trauma-related issues; responding to Oklahoma City; training Israeli and Palestinian mental health practitioners to be EMDR facilitators and/or consultants and hearing their stories; meeting and working with trauma survivors of terrorist attacks in Jerusalem and Bethlehem; seeing the trauma symptoms displayed by Israeli supervisees during a supervisory course and working with their traumas after the second intifada; debriefing with the Philadelphia-based FBI group who responded to 9/11; assisting the friends and relatives of a friend after the brutal murder of his adolescent daughter; attending conferences where disaster responses were emphasized; interviewing 61 members of the EMDR community for the EMDRIA newsletter and hearing about their lives and how they have responded to many different types of disasters (i.e., hurricanes, earthquakes, terrorist attacks, war, acid attacks, etc.) in many different places (i.e., Oklahoma City, Bangladesh, New York, Serbia, Croatia,

Rwanda, Mexico, etc.); and talking and connecting with many more colleagues and friends after they returned from disaster responses.

In 2009, *Eye Movement Desensitization and Reprocessing (EMDR) Scripted Protocols: Basics and Special Situations* (Luber, 2009a) was published. Although it was not a book about recent trauma per se, it did contain at least 10 out of 35 chapters that were recent-trauma related. Clearly, recent trauma was occupying this author's thoughts. This interest in recent trauma was amplified after a presentation at the EMDR European Annual Conference in Amsterdam. Konuk (2009, June) was presenting on "Mental Health Response and Training Program for Developing Countries: Turkish Model." The depth and breadth of his response to this enormous natural disaster was inspiring and seemed an important model that other EMDR disaster responders would be interested to know about. This ongoing Turkish Project began with the response to the earthquake but was continuing currently, and he discussed the elements that he thought were pertinent to a disaster response: financing, the training of mental health professionals, providing psychological services, creating a trauma therapy center, building a trauma library, preparing for other disasters by engaging consultants who had experience in this area, and research. From 1999 until the time of the presentation (2009), his group trained 550 therapists in the EMDR Basic Training. They also trained 900 students and professionals in early trauma intervention skills. In the aftermath of their 1999 disaster project, the response teams have learned so much and are so well organized that they can be on-site within 30 to 60 minutes after any disaster in many areas in Turkey. As a result, they are held in high regard nationally and have had the ability to respond to more earthquakes, floods, bombings, and an airplane crash. Emre's pithy final words were the following, *"If you intend to go into the 'disaster business' in a developing country: Find the owner; find the money; teach organizational skills; teach how to write a proposal; and teach project management!"*

However, it was after the 2011 Tohoku earthquake and tsunami in Japan occurred that the need for this type of book became pressing. This author had visited Japan less than a year before the catastrophe to do an EMDR HAP Military training with Nancy Errebo at the Atsugi Naval Base several hours outside of Tokyo. In the hopes of supporting interaction between the EMDR Japan Association members and the American EMDR-trained mental health personnel on the U.S. military bases in Japan, this author made the formal introductions so that they could get to know and work with each other. When the disaster struck, we were all in touch with each other trying to find ways to support our Japanese colleagues. This author began to pull together the recent trauma-related protocols for our Japanese colleagues and helped them connect with other EMDR practitioners who were experts in the field of recent trauma—all of whom are represented in this book. It became clear that it would be far easier if all of these protocols were housed in one text and/or on a CD version; it was at that point that this author approached her editor at Springer Publishing Company, Sheri W. Sussman, with the idea. However, it was not just the protocols that were of importance; it was also how members of the EMDR community were responding to disasters globally. A proposal was written and accepted.

Implementing EMDR Early Mental Health Interventions for Man-Made and Natural Disasters: Models, Scripted Protocols, and Summary Sheets is akin to the structure in the other EMDR Scripted Protocol texts:

- *Eye Movement Desensitization and Reprocessing (EMDR) Scripted Protocols: Basics and Special Situations* (Luber, 2009a)
- *Eye Movement Desensitization and Reprocessing (EMDR) Scripted Protocols: Special Populations* (Luber, 2009b)
- *Eye Movement Desensitization and Reprocessing (EMDR) Scripted Protocols With Summary Sheets (CD-ROM Version)*: Basics and Special Situations (Luber, 2012a)
- *Eye Movement Desensitization and Reprocessing (EMDR) Scripted Protocols With Summary Sheets (CD-ROM Version): Special Populations* (Luber, 2012b)

The only exception to this structure is the inclusion of the first section on Early Mental Health Intervention Response: An International Perspective.

The following description from *Eye Movement Desensitization and Reprocessing (EMDR) Scripted Protocols: Basics and Special Situations* gives a clear understanding of the evolution and importance of this format:

> *Eye Movement Desensitization and Reprocessing (EMDR) Scripted Protocols: Basics and Special Situations* grew out of a perceived need that mental health practitioners could be served by a place to access both traditional and newly developed protocols in a way that adheres to best clinical practices incorporating the Standard EMDR Protocol that includes working on the past, present, and future issues (the 3-Pronged Protocol) related to the problem and the 11-Step Standard Procedure that includes attention to the following steps: image, negative cognition (NC), positive cognition (PC), validity of cognition (VoC), emotion, subjective units of disturbance (SUD), and location of body sensation, desensitization, installation, body scan, and closure. Often, EMDR texts embed the protocols in a great deal of explanatory material that is essential in the process of learning EMDR. However, sometimes, as a result, practitioners move away from the basic importance of maintaining the integrity of the Standard EMDR Protocol and keeping adaptive information processing in mind when conceptualizing the course of treatment for a patient. It is in this way that the efficacy of this powerful methodology is lost.
>
> "Scripting" becomes a way not only to inform and remind the EMDR practitioner of the component parts, sequence, and language used to create an effective outcome, but it also creates a template for practitioners and researchers to use for reliability and/or a common denominator so that the form of working with EMDR is consistent. The concept that has motivated this work was conceived within the context of assisting EMDR clinicians in accessing the scripts of the full protocols in one place and to profit from the creativity of other EMDR clinicians who have kept the spirit of EMDR but have also taken into consideration the needs of the population with whom they work or the situations that they encounter. Reading a script is by no means a substitute for adequate training, competence, clinical acumen, and integrity; if you are not a trained EMDR therapist and/or you are not knowledgeable in the field for which you wish to use the script, these scripts are not for you.
>
> As EMDR is a fairly complicated process, and indeed, has intimidated some from integrating it into their daily approach to therapy, this book provides step-by-step scripts that will enable beginning practitioners to enhance their expertise more quickly. . . .
>
> These scripted protocols are intended for clinicians who have read Shapiro's text (2001) and received EMDR training from an EMDR-accredited trainer. An EMDR trainer is a licensed mental health practitioner who has been approved by the association active in the clinician's country of practice. (Luber, 2009a, p. xxi)

In 2012, the CD-ROM versions of the original 2009 books were published in a different format. Included in the CD-ROM were just the protocols and summary sheets (the notes were not included and are in the 2009 texts). As explained in the Preface of *Eye Movement Desensitization and Reprocessing (EMDR) Scripted Protocols With Summary Sheets (CD-ROM Version): Basics and Special Situations* (Luber, 2012a):

> The idea for *Eye Movement Desensitization and Reprocessing (EMDR) Scripted Protocols: Summary Sheets for Basics and Special Situations* grew out of the day-to-day work with the protocols that allowed for a deeper understanding of case conceptualization from an EMDR perspective. While using the scripted protocols and acquiring a greater familiarity with the use of the content, the idea of placing the information in a summarized format grew. This book of scripted protocols and summary sheets was undertaken so that clinicians could easily use the material in Eye Movement Desensitization and Reprocessing (EMDR) Scripted Protocols: Basics and Special Situations. While working on the summary sheets, the interest in brevity collided with the thought that clinicians could also use these summary sheets to remind themselves of the steps in the process clarified in the scripted protocols. The original goal to be a summary of the necessary data gathered from the protocol was transformed into this new creation of data summary and memory tickler for the protocol itself! Alas, the summary sheets have become a bit longer than originally anticipated. Nonetheless, they are shorter—for the most part—than the protocols themselves and do summarize the data in an easily readable format. . . .
>
> The format for this book is also innovative. The scripts and summary sheets are available in an expandable, downloadable format for easy digital access. Because EMDR is a fairly complicated process, and often intimidating, these scripted protocols with their accompanying summary sheets can be helpful in a number of ways. To begin with, by facilitating the gathering of

important data from the protocol about the client, the scripted protocol and/or summary sheet then can be inserted into the client's chart as documentation. The summary sheet can assist the clinician in formulating a concise and clear treatment plan with clients and can be used to support quick retrieval of the essential issues and experiences during the course of treatment. Practitioners can enhance their expertise more quickly by having a place that instructs and reminds them of the essential parts of EMDR practice. By having these fill-in PDF forms, clinicians can easily tailor the scripted protocols and summary sheets to the needs of their clients, their consultees/supervisees, and themselves by editing and saving the protocol scripts and summary sheets.

Consultants/Supervisors will find these scripted protocols and summary sheets useful while working with consultees/supervisees in their consultation/supervision groups. These works bring together many ways of handling current, important issues in psychotherapy and EMDR treatment. They also include a helpful way to organize the data collected that is key to case consultation and the incorporation of EMDR into newly trained practitioners' practices. (Luber, 2012a, p. iv)

This main book is divided into eight parts with 26 chapters that include working with recent trauma models of response, resources, on-site responses, individuals, groups, special populations, special situations, and clinician self-care. The first part is devoted to the "Early Mental Health Intervention Response: An International Perspective." There are six chapters included in this section and all of them revolve around how disaster struck in the authors' environments and how they responded. Alan Cohen and Mooli Lahad explain the evolution of their Community Stress Prevention Center (CSPC) that was destined to become one of the earliest (1979)—if not *the* earliest—center to work with a mental health response in Israel and possibly in the world. Through the efforts of the CSPC, many people globally have learned how to respond to major disasters. Their influence is illustrated in the chapters from Turkey and Spain that follow. The second chapter is by Emre Konuk and his assistant, Zeynep Zat. As described above, Emre was part of the Turkish Psychological initiative to respond to the Marmara earthquake of 1999. They describe how, from the beginning, they incorporated a structure upon which they could improve their mental health disaster response capabilities over the years and then explain how they have gone on to accomplish it. Maria Cervera has been one of the major critical incident leaders in Spain. She describes how the Spanish psychologists—with the help of what they learned from Mooli Lahad's CSPC and the Independent Counseling and Advisory Services (ICAS)—built a national network of psychological professionals who are trained in mental health disaster response and related treatments. She explains a number of different interventions and how their ability to respond has made a difference throughout Spain. Ignacio (Nacho) Jarero and Susana Uribe take the opportunity in their chapter to describe Nacho's, "The Seven Phase Model." They describe this multicomponent model for an early psychological intervention program that is carried out by the Early Psychological Intervention Team (EPIT). They discuss in detail what to do before, during, and after deployment to the disaster zone. Through their organization, Asociación Mexicana Para Ayuda Mental en Crisis (AMAMECRISIS), they have assisted and taught their method to many clinicians. The fruits of their work—the Butterfly Hug, the EMDR Integrative Group Treatment Protocol (IGTP) for Children and for Adults, and the EMDR Protocol for Recent Critical Incidents (EMDR-PRECI)—are the gifts from them that we use all around the world. Carol Martin, the Executive Director of EMDR Humanitarian Assistance Programs (EMDR HAP), and Nancy Simons, Clinical Director of EMDR HAP, have written about the lessons learned by this program over the years. They go into more depth about the Trauma Recovery Networks (TRNs) that are forming across the United States to respond to local disasters in their communities and sometimes join other communities, if a response is needed. The last chapter in this part speaks to how a small group of volunteers from Mumbai were able to mount a huge response after the Gujarat earthquake of 2001. Sushma Mehrotra, Mrinalini Purandare, Parul Tank, and Hvovi Bhagwagar discuss this project and what they learned about responding to a major disaster. They, too, created an EMDR group protocol to respond to the needs of the victims.

The second part is devoted to "EMDR Early Mental Health Resources." Although there were many to choose from, there are only two of the most used resources in this section:

the Butterfly Hug created by Luci Artigas and the Four Elements Exercise for Stress Management by Elan Shapiro. These two individuals have been central to the creation of a number of the chapters in this text, as a result of their sensitivity, creativity, and ability to transform a difficult situation by creating something totally new and specific to their context; they truly have the gift of turning therapy into an art form. "EMDR On-Site or Hospital Response" is the third section. In these chapters, we find very resourceful ways to work with trauma victims in the immediacy of their trauma. Gary Quinn's Emergency Response Procedure (ERP) gives us an important way to stabilize patients in the emergency room or on-site. Judith Guedalia's work assisted by Frances Yoeli is called the EMDR Emergency Room and Wards Protocol (EMDR-ER©), and they walk us through a thoughtful way of helping stabilize trauma survivors and creating new narratives for their trauma patients.

The fourth part, "EMDR Early Intervention Procedures for Individuals," presents the scripted protocol for Francine Shapiro's Protocol for Recent Traumatic Events, discussed in the beginning of this Preface. It is the basis—along with the Standard EMDR Protocol—upon which we have constructed our EMDR response for recent trauma. Elan Shapiro and Brurit Laub build on this foundation with their Recent Traumatic Episode Protocol (R-TEP) and help us conceptualize Early EMDR Intervention (EEI). Nacho Jarero and Luci Artigas end this section with their EMDR Protocol for Recent Critical Incidents (EMDR-PRECI). They, too, modify the Protocol for Recent Traumatic Events to incorporate the needs of the victims with whom they work.

"EMDR Early Intervention for Groups" is the subject of the fifth part. The first chapter is the ubiquitous, EMDR Integrative Group Treatment Protocol (IGTP) for Children and the second chapter is a newer version of the IGTP modified for adults. The IGTP has been the basis for group treatment since its inception in the late '90s and has been used around the world. The Imma EMDR Group Protocol by Brurit Laub and Esti Bar-Sade is a modification of the IGTP and offers some interesting and dynamic changes for working with children. Aiton Birnbaum is another creative individual who brought his talents to introducing a workbook format for EMDR. This new approach can be used with individuals or groups and can be helpful especially for those clients who are more visual. It also offers an option for a more private way of working with traumatic material. In this chapter, you will find an actual workbook that you can copy or print out for each client.

First responders are our society's designated protectors. Whether they are firefighters, emergency medical service professionals, the police, or the military, they are trained to respond when many of us would run in the other direction. In the first chapter of Part VI, "EMDR Early Mental Health Interventions: First Responders," Robbie Adler-Tapia delves into the world of first responders/protective service workers including firefighters and emergency medical services (EMS) professionals and helps us understand what we need to know to work with this population. Roger Solomon has been working with the police and law enforcement in many different capacities throughout the course of his career. He blends his knowledge of EMDR with his experience of the police to help us understand what we need to know to work with these officers of the law. Mark Russell is retired from the military with 26 years of service. He has translated his experience, with the help of his assistant, Tammera Cooke, and his colleague, Susan Rogers, a long-time provider of treatment to war and trauma survivors, to introduce us to the world of military. All of these chapters introduce modifications when working with EMDR to accommodate the needs of first responders.

Part VII concerns "EMDR Early Intervention for Special Situations." The first chapter by David Blore is a protocol that addresses the particular issues regarding underground trauma. With his experience working with miners, David helps us enter into their domain so that we have a better appreciation for what the underground world is like and how to approach it when trauma strikes. The next chapter, which David wrote with Manda Holmshaw, grew out of his experience with clients who were uncomfortable revealing the content of their traumas and concerns. Through the EMDR "Blind to Therapist Protocol," they help clients reprocess their material with privacy and dignity.

The last section in the book, Part VII, "EMDR and Clinician Self-Care: Recent Trauma Response," is at the heart of any well-designed disaster response. It is often the case that we take better care of our clients than ourselves. When it comes to disaster response, this attitude can be another type of disaster in the making. Neal Daniels's chapter discusses how we can inoculate ourselves against burnout and secondary PTSD by taking care to process residual material from our work on a regular basis. In Karen Alter-Reid's chapter about her own FR-TRN response to the Newtown shooting tragedy, self-care is a primary ingredient in the organization of their work. There are a number of checks and support systems that create a holding environment for the team so that no one slips through the cracks to face the aftermath of disaster response alone. Derek Farrell responded to the call for facilitators and volunteers to assist in Turkey after the earthquake. His chapter teaches us about how even the most perceptive of clinicians can miss something in the face of such overwhelming destruction. Derek teaches us the signs and symptoms of vicarious trauma and then uses this knowledge to create better caretaking for himself and his clients. The last chapter in this section and the book is about the worst case scenarios in recent trauma response. Nacho and Susana again use the format that they did in Chapter 4 of pre-, during, and post-deployment to create checklists to assure that you have thought of all the variables when responding to disaster.

Appendix A includes the scripts for the 3-Pronged Protocol that includes past memories, current triggers, and future templates. These scripts are there to assist practitioners so that they can place them in clients' charts to use with a particular issue or as a reminder of all of the elements needed for the work to be complete.

Appendix B is an updated list of all of the EMDR associations and regional associations globally. In this way, it is possible to know where practitioners of EMDR are to be found in any part of the world. This list also includes the EMDR Humanitarian Assistance Programs that exist to help victims of man-made and natural disasters. There are also resources that catalogue information such as the Francine Shapiro Library, an invaluable source of knowledge for any EMDR practitioner. There are also links to the *EMDR Journal* and other e-journals where trauma-related information can be found.

This book is meant to go with you to disasters. Here, you will find a great deal of information that will support you in responding to the challenges that you might face when designing a disaster response or responding to a disaster. Each one of these protocols has been tried in the field. Although there is no definitive research about them, it has begun to trickle in, and you can be the next author of research in this area. Try these suggestions and protocols in your own community and join your Humanitarian Assistance Program groups and/or TRNs to create an EMDR disaster response that is felt around the world.

REFERENCES

Aduriz, M. E., Knopfler, C., & Bluthgen, C. (2009). Helping child flood victims using group EMDR intervention in Argentina: Treatment outcome and gender differences. *International Journal of Stress Management, 16,* 138–153.

Altan Aytun, O., Ozcan, G., Ciftci, A,. Konuk, E. Yuksek, H., Karakus, D., . . . Vatan Ozcelik, D. (2010, June). The effects of early EMDR interventions (EMD and R-TEP) on the victims of a terrorist bombing in Istanbul. In *Treatment of children/acute stress*. Symposium conducted at the annual meeting of the EMDR Europe Association, Hamburg, Germany.

American Psychiatric Association (APA). (2004). *Practice guideline for the treatment of patients with acute stress disorder and posttraumatic stress disorder.* Arlington, VA: American Psychiatric Association Practice Guidelines.

Andrews, B., Brewin, C. R., Philpott, R., & Stewart, L. (2007). Delayed-onset posttraumatic stress disorder: A systematic review of the evidence. *American Journal of Psychiatry, 164*(9), 1319–1326.

Artigas, L., Jarero, I., Mauer, M., López Cano, T., & Alcalá, N. (2000, September). *EMDR and traumatic stress after natural disasters: Integrative treatment protocol and the Butterfly Hug.* Poster presented at the EMDRIA Conference, Toronto, Ontario, Canada.

Artigas, L., Jarero, I., Alcalá, N., & Lopez-Cano, T. (2009). The EMDR Integrative Group Treatment Protocol (IGTP). In M. Luber (Ed.) *Eye movement desensitization and reprocessing (EMDR) scripted protocols: Basic and special situations* (pp. 279–288). New York, NY: Springer.

Australian Centre for Posttraumatic Mental Health. (2007). *Australian Guidelines for the Treatment of Adults with Acute Stress Disorder and Posttraumatic Stress Disorder.* Melbourne, Victoria: Author.

Bleich, A., Kotler, M., Kutz, I., & Shalev, A. (2002). *Guidelines for the assessment and professional intervention with terror victims in the hospital and in the community.* A position paper of the (Israeli) National Council for Mental Health, Jerusalem, Israel.

Bryant, R. A., Friedman, M. J., Spiegel, D., Ursano, R., & Strain. J. (2010). A review of acute stress disorder in *DSM-5. Depression and Anxiety, 28*(9), 802–817.

Bryant, R. A., Creamer, M., O'Donnell, M., Silove, D., & McFarlane, A. C. (2011). The capacity of acute stress disorder to predict posttraumatic psychiatric disorders. *Journal of Psychiatric Research, 46*(2), 168–173.

California Evidence-Based Clearinghouse for Child Welfare. (2010). *Trauma treatment for children.* Retrieved from www.cebc4cw.org

Chambless, D. L., Baker, M. J., Baucom, D. H., Beutler, L. E., Calhoun, K. S., Cris-Christoph, P., . . . Woody, S. R. (1998). Update on empirically validated therapies, II. *The Clinical Psychologist, 51,* 3–16.

Chemtob, C. M., Tolin, D. F., van der Kolk, B. A., & Pitman, R. K. (2000). Eye movement desensitization and reprocessing. In E. A. Foa, T. M. Keane, & M. J. Friedman (Eds.). *Effective treatments for PTSD: Practice guidelines from the International Society for Traumatic Stress Studies.* New York, NY: Guilford.

Clinical Resource Efficiency Support Team. (2003). *The management of posttraumatic stress disorder in adults.* A publication of the Clinical Resource Efficiency Support Team of the Northern Ireland Department of Health, Social Services and Public Safety, Belfast.

Colelli, G., & Patterson, B. (2008). Three case reports illustrating the use of the protocol for recent traumatic events following the World Trade Center terrorist attack. *Journal of EMDR Practice and Research, 2*(2), 114–123.

Department of Veterans Affairs and Department of Defense. (2004). *VA/DoD clinical practice guideline for the management of post-traumatic stress.* Washington, DC: Veterans Health Administration, Department of Veterans Affairs and Health Affairs, Department of Defense. Office of Quality and Performance publication 10Q-CPG/PTSD-04.

Dutch National Steering Committee Guidelines Mental Health Care. (2003). Multidisciplinary Guideline Anxiety Disorders. Utrecht, Netherlands: Quality Institute Health Care CBO/Trimbos Institute.

Errebo, N., Knipe, J., Forte, K., Karlin, V., & Altayli, B. (2008). EMDR-HAP training in Sri Lanka following 2004 tsunami. *Journal of EMDR Practice & Research, Fernandez (2002) 2*(2), 124–139.

Fernandez, I. (2002, Dicembre). I disturbi post-traumatici da stress Fattori di rischio, aspetti diagnostici e trattamento con l'EMDR (The post-traumatic stress disorder factors of risk, diagnostic aspects and treatment with the EMDR). Rivista Scientifica di Psicologia, Sommario 01, 15–124.

Fernandez, I. (2007). EMDR as treatment of post-traumatic reactions: A field study on children victims of an earthquake. *Educational and Child Psychology, 24*(1), 65–72.

Fernandez, I. (2008). EMDR after a critical incident: treatment of a tsunami survivor with acute posttraumatic disorder. *Journal of EMDR Practice and Research, 2*(2), 156–159.

Fernandez, I., Gallinari, E., & Lorenzetti, A. (2004). A school-based intervention for children who witnessed the Pirelli building airplane crash in Milan, Italy. *Journal of Brief Therapy, 2,* 129–136.

Foa, E. B. (2009). *Effective treatments for PTSD: Practice guidelines from the International Society for Traumatic Stress Studies,* 2nd ed. New York, NY: Guilford.

Gelbach, R., & Davis, K. (2007). Disaster response: EMDR and family systems therapy under community-wide stress. In F. Shapiro, F. W. Kaslow, & L. Maxfield (Eds.), *Handbook of EMDR and family therapy processes* (pp. 387–406). New York, NY: John Wiley.

Grainger, R. D., Levin, C., Allen-Byrd, L., Doctor, R. M., & Lee, H. (1997). An empirical evaluation of eye movement desensitization and reprocessing (EMDR) with survivors of a natural disaster. *Journal of Traumatic Stress, 10,* 665–671.

Ichii, M., & Kumano, H. (1996). Application of eye movement desensitization (EMD) to the acute stress disorder victims suffered from the Great Hanshin-Awaji Earthquake. *Japanese Journal of Brief Psychotherapy, 5,* 53–68.

Ichii, M., & Kumano, H. (1996). Eye movement desensitization by Kobe earthquake victims with acute stress disorder (EMD) application. *Japanese Association of Brief Psychotherapy, Research Brief, 5,* 53–70.

INSERM. (2004). *Psychotherapy: An evaluation of three approaches.* Paris, France: French National Institute of Health and Medical Research.

Jarero, I., & Artigas, L. (2010). The EMDR Integrative Group Treatment Protocol: Application with adults during ongoing geopolitical crisis. *Journal of EMDR Practice and Research, 4*(4), 148–155

Jarero, I., Artigas, L., & Hartung, J. (2006). EMDR Integrative Group Treatment Protocol: A post-disaster trauma intervention for children and adults. *Traumatology, 12,* 121–129.

Jarero, I., Artigas, L., & Luber, M. (2011). The EMDR Protocol for Recent Critical Incidents: Application in a disaster mental health continuum of care context. *Journal of EMDR Practice and Research, 5*(3), 82–94.

Jarero, I., Artigas, L., Mauer, M., López Cano, T., & Alcalá, N. (1999, November). *Children's post traumatic stress after natural disasters: Integrative treatment protocol.* Poster presented at the annual meeting of the International Society for Traumatic Stress Studies, Miami, Florida.

Jarero, I., Artigas, L, & Montero, M. (2008). The EMDR Integrative Group Treatment Protocol: Application with child victims of mass disaster. *Journal of EMDR Practice & Research, 2*(2), 97–105.

Jarero, I., & Uribe, S. (2011). The EMDR Protocol for Recent Critical Incidents: Brief report of an application in a human massacre situation. *Journal of EMDR Practice and Research, 5*(4), 156–165.

Jarero, I., & Uribe, S. (2012). The EMDR Protocol for Recent Critical Incidents: Follow-up report of an application in a human massacre situation. *Journal of EMDR Practice and Research, 6*(2), 50–61

Korkmazlar-Oral, U., & Pamuk, S. (2002). Group EMDR with child survivors of the earthquake in Turkey. *Journal of the American Academy of Child and Adolescent Psychiatry, 37*, 47–50.

Konuk, E. (June, 2009). *Mental Health Response and Training Program for Developing Countries: Turkish Model*. Paper presented at the EMDR Europe Association Conference, Amsterdam.

Kutz, I., Resnick, V., & Dekel R. (2008). The effect of single-session modified EMDR on acute stress syndromes. *Journal of EMDR Practice and Research, 2*(3), 190–200

Laub, B., & Bar-Sade, E. (2009a). In M. Luber (Ed.), *Eye movement desensitization and reprocessing (EMDR) scripted protocols: Basics and special situations*. New York, NY: Springer.

Luber, M. (2009b) (Ed.). *Eye movement desensitization and reprocessing (EMDR) scripted protocols: Special populations*. New York, NY: Springer.

Luber, M. (2012a) (Ed.). *Eye movement desensitization and reprocessing (EMDR) scripted protocols with summary sheets (CD-Rom version): Basics and special situations*. New York, NY: Springer.

Luber, M. (2012b) (Ed.). *Eye movement desensitization and reprocessing (EMDR) scripted protocols with summary sheets (CD-Rom version): Special populations*. New York, NY: Springer.

McFarlane, A. C. (2010a). *Abstract to plenary presentation*. Paper presented at EMDR Europe Annual Conference, Hamburg, Germany.

McFarlane, A. C. (2010b). The long-term costs of traumatic stress: intertwined physical and psychological consequences. *World Psychiatry, 9*, 3–10.

Maxfield, L. (2008). EMDR treatment of recent events and community disasters. *Journal of EMDR Practice & Research, 2*(2), 74–78.

National Collaborating Centre for Mental Health. (2005). *Post traumatic stress disorder (PTSD): The management of adults and children in primary and secondary care*. London, England: National Institute for Clinical Excellence.

National Institute for Clinical Excellence (2005, March). *Post-traumatic stress (PTSD): The management of PTSD in adults and children and secondary care*. London, England: National Collaborating Centre for Mental Health.

Roberts, N. P., Kitchiner, N. J., Kenardy, J., & Bisson, J. I. (2009). Multiple session early psychological interventions for the prevention of post-traumatic stress disorder. The Cochrane Library (Issue 3). [DOI: 10.1002/14651858.CD006869.pub2].

Roberts, N. P., Kitchiner, N. J., Kenardy, J., & Bisson, J. I. (2009). Systematic review and meta-analysis of multiple-session early interventions following traumatic events. *American Psychiatric Association, AJP in Advance*. Retrieved fromajp.psychiatryonline.org

Russell, M. C. (2006). Treating combat-related stress disorders: Multiple case study utilizing eye movement desensitization and reprocessing (EMDR) with battlefield casualties from the Iraqi war. *Military Psychology, 18*, 1–18.

SAMHSA's National Registry of Evidence-based Programs and Practices. (2011). Retrieved from http://nrepp.samhsa.gov/ViewIntervention.aspx?id = 199

Schubert, S., & Lee, C. W. (2009). Adult PTSD and its treatment with EMDR: A review of controversies, evidence, and theoretical knowledge. *Journal of EMDR Practice and Research, 3*(3), 117–132.

Shapiro, E. (2009). EMDR treatment of recent trauma. *Journal of EMDR Practice and Research, 3*(3), 141–151.

Shapiro, E. (2012, October). EMDR and early psychological intervention following trauma. *European Review of Applied Psychology, 62*(4), 241–251.

Shapiro, E., & Fernandez, I. (2013, June). *Early EMDR intervention (EEI): Theory, practice and research application in a mass disaster*. Presentation at the annual meeting of the EMDR Europe Association, Geneva, Switzerland.

Shapiro, E., & Laub, B. (2008). Early EMDR intervention (EEI): A summary, a theoretical model, and the recent traumatic episode protocol (R-TEP). *Journal of EMDR Practice and Research, 2*(2), 79–96

Shapiro, F. (1989). Eye movement desensitization: A new treatment model for post-traumatic stress disorder. *Journal of Behavior Therapy and Experimental Psychiatry, 20*, 211–217.

Shapiro, F. (1991). Eye movement desensitization and reprocessing procedure: From EMD to EMDR-a new treatment model for anxiety and related traumata. *Behavior Therapist, 14*, 122–125.

Shapiro, F. (1995) *Eye movement desensitization and reprocessing: Basic principles, protocols and procedures*. New York, NY: Guilford Press.

Shapiro, F. (2001). *Eye movement desensitization and reprocessing: Basic principles, protocols and procedures*. 2nd ed.New York, NY: Guilford Press.

Shapiro, F. (2004). *Military and post-disaster response manual*. Hamden, CT: EMDR Humanitarian Assistance Program.

Shapiro, F. (2006). *EMDR: New notes on adaptive information processing with case formulation principles, forms, scripts and worksheets*. Watsonville, CA: EMDR Institute.

Shapiro, F., Kaslow, F. W., & Maxfield, L. (2007). *Handbook of EMDR and family therapy processes*. Hoboken, NJ: Wiley.

Silver, S. M., Rogers, S., Knipe, J., & Colelli, G. (2005, February). EMDR therapy following the 9/11 terrorist attacks: A community-based intervention project in New York City. *International Journal of Stress Management, 12*(1), 29–42.

Sjöblom, P. O., Andréewitch, S., Bejerot, S., Mörtberg, E., Brinck, U., Ruck, C., & Körlin, D. (2003). *Regional treatment recommendation for anxiety disorders*. Stockholm, Sweden: Medical Program Committee/Stockholm

Therapy Advisor (2004–2007), Retrieved from www.therapyadvisor.com

Tofani, L. R., & Wheeler, K. (2012). Le protocole de l'épisode traumatique récent: Evaluation et analyse des résultats de trois études de cas [The protocol for recent traumatic episode: Evaluation and analysis of the results of three case studies]. *Journal of EMDR Practice and Research, 6*(4), 46E–63E.

United Kingdom Department of Health. (2001). *Treatment choice in psychological therapies and counselling evidence based clinical practice guideline*. London, England: Author.

U.S. Department of Veterans Affairs, Veterans Health Administration & Department of Defense. (2004, January). VA/DoD clinical practice guideline for the management of post-traumatic stress. Version 1.0. Washington, DC: Veterans Health Administration, and Department of Defense.

Vanitallie, T. B. (2002). Stress: A risk factor for serious illness. *Metabolism, 51*(6 Suppl. 1), 40–45.

Wesson, M., & Gould, M. (2009). Intervening early with EMDR on military operations. *Journal of EMDR Practice and Research, 3*(2), 91–97.

Wilson, S., Tinker, R., Hofmann, A., Becker, L., & Marshall, S. (2000). *A field study of EMDR with Kosovar-Albanian refugee children using a group treatment protocol*. Paper presented at the annual meeting of the International Society for the Study of Traumatic Stress, San Antonio, TX.

Zaghrout-Hodali, M., Alissa, F., & Dodgson, P. (2008). Building resilience and dismantling fear: EMDR group protocol with children in an area of ongoing trauma. *Journal of EMDR Practice & Research, 2*(2), 106–113.

Acknowledgments

As a young girl and on into my adolescence, I had the good fortune to grow up in an international community. In this oasis of the International School of Geneva (Ecolint) and under the greater global community fostered by the many international organizations that were headquartered there, I lived in a place where we all coexisted in a type of harmony that—it turns out—is rare. Our school community had its wrinkles but the bullying and the rage that one hears so frequently now, at least to me, was not apparent. We learned to think and reason and negotiate. Through our Students' United Nations, we fought the battles of our world through words and compromise. Simply put, we all got along with each other and if we had a problem, we worked it out. My first year of college shattered that pristine experience of cooperation and tolerance; it was 1968 and the end of my first year when the streets of Paris erupted and chaos ensued as "La revolution de mai" held the whole city hostage. Returning to the States in the middle of the Vietnam War opened my eyes to the fact that the lessons that I learned in Geneva were certainly not happening where I found myself and I discovered later that my friends from Ecolint felt that same way. Since then, I have learned a great deal about trauma and, sadly, it is everywhere.

I would like to acknowledge the need for us—as an EMDR international community—to be part of an initiative to turn this state of affairs around. This book, *Implementing EMDR Early Mental Health Interventions for Man-Made and Natural Disasters: Models, Scripted Protocols, and Summary Sheets*, is an attempt to help my colleagues in the EMDR community learn more about what is needed to respond in the face of disaster and help victims heal and reclaim their lives.

I had two major experiences that pushed me toward the formulation of this book: hearing Emre Konuk present and the 2011 Tōhoku earthquake and tsunami in Japan. First, I would like to acknowledge my friend and colleague, Emre Konuk. It was Emre's presentation at the 2009 EMDR Europe Conference on the Turkish Model for a mental health response that inspired me to learn more about disaster response. As I got to know Emre better through attending conferences and a trip to Turkey, I heard more and more about the breadth and depth of his projects and felt that his gift of organization and creating projects for the greater good was information that we all needed to access.

The 2011 disaster in Japan was of a more personal nature for me. I first traveled to Japan in 1976 with my parents, who had a small business selling Japanese prints. I opened a Japanese art gallery that same year with my father and for a short time I ran the gallery before I decided to go back to teaching and then become a clinical psychologist. The gallery continued and the walls of my world have literally been filled with the aesthetic of Japan since then. I have been back several more times since my first trip for personal, art, and EMDR-related work.

I would like to acknowledge the work of Masaya Ichii who—in fact—was one of the first to use EMD with earthquake survivors after the 1995 Kobe earthquake. Masaya has gone on to become a trainer and create J-HAP, and has been an important force in helping EMDR develop in Japan. I would also like to acknowledge Shigeyuki Ota who did much to support the Japanese response in Tōhoku, as well as Elan Shapiro, Brurit Laub, Nacho Jarero, Masamichi Honda, Kiwamu Tanaka, Masako Kitamura, Robert Gelbach, Derek Farrell, Sushma Mehrotra, Richard Smith, Emre Konuk, Miyako Shirakawa, Akiko Kikuchi,

Keisuki Niki, Pam Brown, Rashid Qayyum, and many other EMDR colleagues from all over the world who helped sustain the EMDR response in Japan.

From the early days of EMDR, Roger Solomon's name was synonymous with working in the area of recent trauma. With his knowledge and experience with the police and other law enforcement agencies, Roger was the person to whom we all went when we had questions concerning early EMDR intervention, critical incident response, and traumatic grief. I would like to acknowledge Roger for all of the work that he has done in this area for all of us in the EMDR community. I would also like to thank you for your support over the years and the grace with which you answered all the questions that I had or assisted me with your insights concerning areas of recent trauma, no matter where you were or what you were doing. Also, for reconnecting me with my old friend, Jim McIntosh, who as an FBI agent helped me understand more clearly the impact of recent trauma and the horrors of 9/11.

I would like us all to remember and celebrate Jim who passed away after his own long battle with illness for his service to his family, friends, and country.

I would like to recognize my friend, Robert Wittman, fellow traveler, FBI agent, and Japanese aficionado who always knows how to climb over any mountain to get to the other side.

There are a number of other people whom I would like to acknowledge concerning this book as it would not have happened without the learning that I gained from our discussions; the hashing out and back and forth of our conversations helped me have a greater appreciation for the nuances of these ideas. To my friends, Elan Shapiro and Brurit Laub, words cannot express how much our discussions have meant to me in the understanding of early EMDR intervention and my respect for your continuing creativity and kindness of spirit. To the three gentleman who underwrote my "trauma fact-finding trip" to Kiryat Schmona (Alan Cohen), Jerusalem (Gary Quinn), and Tel Aviv (Udi Oren) to help me understand the impact of recent trauma and find ways to raise money for more EMDR trainings in the Middle East. To all of the consultants who attended the many consultancy trainings that we (often with Elan) created together in Israel—your willingness to share the innermost parts of yourselves during our work together created a profound learning experience that touched me deeply.

I would like to acknowledge Nacho Jarero, Lucy Artigas, and Susana Uribe, a braver group of people I cannot imagine. Thank you for your friendship and the joy that you take in the most simple of pleasures, even as you go into "battle" or put on your hazmat suits. I have learned more about the spirit that one needs to face the evils of the world and come out on the other side well and—always—with the "Ministry of Presence."

I would like to acknowledge the strength and heart of my female friends and colleagues: Lucy Artigas, Sushma Mehrotra, Mona Zaghrout, Maria Cervera, Robbie Dunton, Rosalie Thomas, Peggy Moore, Susanna Uribe, Kerstin Bergh Johannesson, Phyllis Klaus, Zara Yellin, Zona Scheiner, Barbara Hensley, Catherine Fine, Irene Geissl, Elaine Alvarez, Barbara Grinnell, Robbie Adler-Tapia, Carolyn Settle, Kate Wheeler, Sandra Wilson, Victoria Britt, Sheila Bender, Marsha Heiman, Delphine Pecoul, Maria Elena Aduriz, Ligia Barascout de Piedra Santa, Louise Maxfield, Joany Spierings, Reyhana Ravat, Jennifer Lendl, Deany Laliotis, Francisca Garcia Guerra, Esly Carvalho, Eva Muenker-Kramer, Nancy Errebo, Luise Reddemann, Phyllis Goltra, Priscilla Marquis, Barbara Parrett, Carlijn de Roos, Linda Cohn, Jocelyne Shiromoto, Christine Rost, Martine Tiedt-Schutte, Elfrun Magloire, Eva Zimmerman, Esther Ebner, France Haour, Hanne Hummel, Shelley Weber, Hope Riley, Brenda Byrne, Veronika Engl, Isabel Fernancez, Sandy Shapiro, Ruth Heber, Ellen Latenstein, Karen Alter Reid, Sue Evans, Susan Schaefer, Lulu Medina, Debby Korn, Brurit Laub, Sandra Wilson, Elizabeth Snyker, Hellen Hornsveld, Renee Beer, Christie Sprowls, Barbara Korzun, Patti Levin, Jocelyn Barrett, Reg Morrow, Carol Crow, Carol Forgash, Esti Bar Sade, Isabelle Meignant, Tessa Prattos, Jenny Ann Rydberg, Fran Yoeli, Katy Murray, Sandra Paulsen, Donna D'Aloia, Katy O'Shea, Sandra Kaplan, Nancy Smith, Dorothy Ashman, Wendy Freitag, Pam Brown, Laurie Tetrault, Ana Gomez, Kay Werk, Debra Wesselmann, Maria Masciandaro, Betsy Prince, Jill Strunk, Denise Gelinas, Sandi Richman, Shelley Uram, Frankie Klaff, Edith Taber, Celia Grand, Cynthia Kong, Blanche Freund, Francine Shapiro, and all of the extraordinary women I have met on this journey.

To Derek Farrell who has become a friend—not just a colleague—over the past several years, I would like to thank you for your ability to keep grounded despite the difficulties around you and for the gift of your experience that you have given to all of us.

To Richard Mitchell, my old friend and fellow voyager on our trip to Bethlehem that opened our eyes and souls. To Jim Knipe who has been a great support. To Bob Gelbach, Howard Wainer, Donald Nathanson, and Stuart Wolfe who have been strong supporters of my writing. To AJ Popky who introduced me to EMDR.

To Steve Silver, I thank you for all that I have learned from you while doing EMDR supervision groups together, for your willingness to answer questions, and for always looking for the "light in the heart of darkness." I would like to acknowledge Susan Rogers and Elaine Alvarez for stepping in at a time that I needed assistance and making everything clear. Thank you also to Elan Shapiro, Brurit Laub, Nacho Jarero, and Roger Solomon for helping when another set of eyes or four was needed.

I would also like to remember Kathy Davis who left us with the legacy of her wisdom, her knowledge, and her kindness.

I would like to thank the Springer staff, especially my editor, Sheri W. Sussman, for her encouragement and support in the face of many demands on my time during this period of writing.

Always, I want to thank and acknowledge you, Francine. Your discovery, your creativity, your persistence, and your ability to open a new door that is EMDR has been one of the greatest gifts in my life and uncountable others.

I am dedicating this book to my mother who has been going through her own recent trauma with the spirit and true determination that she has always displayed throughout her life; a role model for us all.

EMDR and Clinician Self-Care: Recent Trauma Response

The mental health profession attracts those of us who want to help. Whether it is working as a school counselor, a community mental health provider, psychiatric inpatient practitioner, supervisor, private practitioner, etc., we hear the siren call of the wounded and the hurting and we run to assist them. In a local context, when we listen to the daily local news about the tragedies of a victim of a drunk driver, a neighborhood torn apart by drug and gun violence, we want to do something. On a larger scale, we see—before our eyes—the terrified and stricken eyes of children from Haiti, Turkey, Serbia, Ethiopia, Newtown (the list goes on and on), as a result of a man-made or natural disaster, and we wonder, "Is there anything that we can do to help?"

There is much that our EMDR community is doing and has been doing in response to these devastating man-made and natural disasters. We mental health practitioners often make the transition to mental health responders in critical incidents with what seems a great deal of ease. However, the underbelly of our wish—if not need—to help, is the question, "At what cost?"

Graduate programs in psychology, social work, and family therapy and medical school programs for physicians, nurse practitioners, and psychiatric nurses rarely, if ever, speak to the needs of the actual students whom they are training. The underlying message is that we are to "soldier through" the difficulties with little thought to our own needs and well-being. Indeed, if we take the time out to breathe or "take a day for ourselves," somehow we are not living up to our credo "to serve."

Early in the EMDR community, we had not yet made the link between self-care and good clinical practice. Many of us, spurred on by the gift and excitement of working with a psychotherapeutic method that actually helped clients heal from deep wounds and trauma, walked, biked, drove, trained, and flew to all parts of the globe to help teach our colleagues everywhere, what we had found to be so effective. In the beginning, many of us traveled almost every weekend—while working at our "day jobs." Over time, we grew more fatigued and began to realize that we needed more balance in our lifestyle. Nowhere was this more apparent than for those of us who responded to the major disasters in places such as Bangladesh, Croatia, China, Colombia, Columbine, Ethiopia, Haiti, Israel, Japan, Lebanon, Mexico, New York, Oklahoma City, Rwanda, South Africa, Turkey, etc.—the list is long. Often, we struggled when we came back, wondering why we were so tired, emotionally exhausted, depressed, not as interested as we had been, or worse still, we just felt that way and were so deeply in it that we did not even wonder at all.

Some of us began early on to use the phenomenon of bilateral stimulation (BLS), introduced by Francine Shapiro. Neal Daniels, the first contributor in this section, paid particular attention to not only his patients' welfare, he was also concerned about his staff and his own response to working at the Philadelphia VA Medical Center. They listened to their patients' daily accounts of horror from the war, about their return From war, the effect of living with disability, and the heavy emotional responses they were having, including the toll that all of these experiences took on themselves and their families. Understanding the nature of vicarious traumatization, Neal asked his staff to use EMDR on their "peskies," as he was doing. His chapter on "Self-Care for EMDR Practitioners" is his way of reminding his team and us about the importance of regular self-care.

Karen Alter-Reid, a humanitarian and exceptional organizer, consented to write a chapter on short notice for this project as she is—at this moment—in the midst of her Trauma Recovery Network (TRN) response by her own newly-formed Fairfield County TRN to the Newtown, Connecticut, tragedy. Her chapter "Community Trauma: A Blueprint for Support and Treatment for Trauma Recovery Network Responders From the Newtown, CT, Tragedy" is a testimony to how far we have come in knowing how important it is to take care of the bodies, minds, and souls of our responders. Her chapter is filled with the wisdom that grew out of a "Therapy for Therapists" project in New Orleans, coordinated by Sue Evans, HAP volunteer, following Hurricanes Katrina and Rita, where colleagues were suffering from "shared traumatic reality" (Baum, 2010). The hallmark of this project was to build resilience for responders, educate them about shared traumatic realities, bring in other clinicians from outside the community to treat them, provide EMDR treatment before giving the on-site therapists Part I of the EMDR Basic Training to optimize learning through the reprocessing of their trauma, and model effective EMDR treatment by seasoned EMDR clinicians. The result of this project informed the way Karen set up this current project.

The next chapter, "Vicarious Trauma and EMDR," is an extraordinary account by a man who has the capacity to look deep inside himself at one of the most difficult times in his life. The stark description of the devastating 1999 Turkish earthquake is penetrating and reveals to us the day-to-day misery behind the headlines that we read online and in the newspapers. Derek Farrell helps us to understand the impact this critical incident had on him and the terrible struggle that ensued as he tried to come to terms with what happened to him over many months, during and after his trip to aid the survivors in Turkey. He looks back and walks us through the symptoms that he better appreciated in retrospect and helps us understand the true nature of what it means to experience and live inside vicarious trauma. As he describes the process of recovering from this ordeal, he teaches us about the importance of looking at trauma from multiple perspectives or narratives. He also gives us a model for thinking about this issue as we work with our own clients. Learning from his experience in Turkey, he continued his humanitarian work—later becoming the President of EMDR Europe HAP—and introduced the idea that a member of the team needs to be responsible for the psychological support of all team members. With this in mind, he created, the "EMDR Positive 'Stay and Go' Group Exercise" so that each team member could acknowledge being part of the team, his/her own contribution, take time to value him/herself, acknowledge his/her individual needs, and participate in a group share/grounding exercise to be done at the end of the team's work. He also recommends follow up with each member of the team post training.

Ignacio Jarero and Susana Uribe wrote the last chapter in this section and in this book. These two colleagues—along with members of their team—have taught this author a great deal about the profound effect of recent trauma on a large scale. They go in to places where many of us would be terrified to go and talk about it candidly. The tales they tell of the work that they have done in the wake of hurricanes, earthquakes, Mexican drug cartels, and massacres can give you the clarity to understand at a deeper level the aftermath and far-reaching consequences of these catastrophes. Perhaps the most disturbing experience for me was when Nacho was in Haiti working for Vision Request after the disastrous earthquake of 2010. Although I had been in contact with him through many of his disaster responses, I had never seen or heard him so shaken. He asked all of his friends and family to keep in contact with him during those dark days so that he could have the virtual knowledge—if he could not have the concrete ability to touch us and look into our eyes—that we were with him.

Working in the aftermath of a disaster is not for the faint of heart, and Nacho and Susana help us understand what we must do to keep safe, sane, and grounded by connecting to ourselves and remembering and linking into what and who bring us sustenance. In their chapter, "Worst Case Scenarios in Recent Trauma Response," they help us to understand our needs before, during, and after deployment. Their insistence on self-care as a seminal part of any structured response is clear and resonates through this chapter. Clear message is this: If you can take care of yourself in the midst of this type of chaos as you give of yourself, the rewards will touch you deep into the core of your being.

During an interview, soon after 9/11, Roger Solomon, an EMDR Trainer and expert in working with law enforcement and critical incidents, was asked, "How have you learned to handle other people's trauma?" He responded with the following:

> How have I learned to handle other people's trauma? It has definitely been a learning experience over the years. It is a continual process of learning to deal with my own vulnerability as I deal with other people's vulnerability. The best way I have found to deal with it is to be part of a team, with colleagues that I trust. We can talk, debrief, and take care of each other. In New York, I am working with other people whom I have worked with for years, and trust. Another important factor is that I see people get better. When I am working with someone who is traumatized, whether it is a police widow or a WTC survivor, my mindset is that his/her current emotional state is normal and temporary. Things will improve, and I will be part of that forward movement and resolution. This keeps my work meaningful and prevents burnout. The efficacy of EMDR has played a significant role in the development of this outlook. (Luber, 2001)

Summary sheets are included to enter data and to provide checklists of important information for your quick retrieval.

Learning how to give service to victims of man-made and natural disasters and to our first responders, police and the military is an important part of any disaster response and key to the vitality of the communities in which we live. By also tending to our own needs, we are able to look after the needs of others and do extraordinary things.

Self-Care for EMDR Practitioners

Neal Daniels

Introduction

This protocol was derived from the notes of Neal Daniels, a clinical psychologist who was the director of the PTSD Clinical Team at the Philadelphia VA Medical Center in Pennsylvania. Always concerned about the welfare of clients and practitioners, he put together a short, simple, and effective protocol for the practitioner, on the completion of any session where there was negative affect remaining.

Self-Care Script Notes

In Neal's words, "The procedure is short, simple, effective. Right after the session or later on in the day when it is possible, bring up the image of the patient; do 10–15 eye movements; generate a positive cognition and install it with the patient's image and another 10–15 movements. Once the negative affects have been reduced, realistic formulations about the patient's future therapy are much easier to develop. Residual feelings of anger, frustration, regret, or hopelessness have been replaced by clearer thoughts about what can or cannot be done. Positive, creative mulling can proceed without the background feelings of unease, weariness, and ineffectiveness. Daily, weekly, or even career-long "burnout" can be viewed as the accumulated residual of negative feelings that were not dealt with effectively when they occurred." The idea was to work on the material right after the session or later in the day when time allowed.

Clinician Self-Care Script

Say, *"Bring up the image of the patient."*

_____

_____

Do 10-15 eye movements

Say, *"Notice whatever positive cognition comes to mind."*

_____

_____

Say, *"Now install the positive cognition_____(state the positive cognition) with the patient's image."*

Do 10–15 eye movements.

Say, *"What do you notice?"*

_____

_____

Once the negative affects have been reduced, realistic formulations about the patient's future therapy are much easier to develop. Residual feelings of anger, frustration, regret, or hopelessness have been replaced by clearer thoughts about what can or cannot be done. Positive, creative mulling can proceed without the background feelings of unease, weariness, and ineffectiveness.

Daily, weekly, or even career-long burnout can be viewed as the accumulated residual of negative feelings that were not dealt with effectively when they occurred.

SUMMARY SHEET:
Self-Care for EMDR Practitioners

1A

Neal Daniels
SUMMARY SHEET BY MARILYN LUBER

Name: _____

   Image of Patient: _____

_____

Image of Patient + BLS

PC that comes up: _____

PC + BLS

Results: _____

_____

_____

To prevent burnout, do after each session.

Community Trauma: A Blueprint for Support and Treatment for Trauma Recovery Network (TRN) Responders From the Newtown, CT, Tragedy

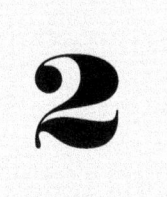

Karen Alter-Reid

Introduction

A devastating fire in Stamford, Connecticut, on Christmas morning 2011 shook our town and took the lives of three young children and their grandparents. We soon learned that the community had no organized mental health response in place to help the first responders after the rescue and recovery efforts. Because it was Christmas Day, agencies were not receiving or responding to emergency calls. Phone calls to some of our EMDR colleagues began to unfold, inviting us to be a presence at a debriefing at the firehouse that week. The fire department was devastated after this horrific fire, beginning with being woken up on Christmas morning to a call that involved children in harm's way. This marked the beginning of the formation of our Stamford Trauma Recovery Network (TRN). Six of our EMDR colleagues treated some of the firemen pro bono as our newly formed team, coordinated by Michael Crouch, LCSW, and myself, met to discuss mission, membership, and structure. We collaborated with HAP for assistance in shaping goals and began to network with the local fire and police departments, offering them traumatology workshops and education about EMDR treatment. Placing mental health clinicians, including our own TRN members, at the top of the list of our definition of "First Responders" was an outgrowth of my involvement in other HAP projects (Alter-Reid, Evans, & Schaefer, 2010). "Shared traumatic reality" (Baum, 2010) is essential to be prepared for, when training or working clinically with first responder therapists in disaster areas. Therefore, our TRN included a chairperson for "Caring for Our Own Therapists."

The Newtown, CT, Shooting TRN Response

When we heard of the Newtown school shooting on December 14, 2012, nearly a year after the Christmas Day fire in Stamford, our TRN was in place and had just been trained two months earlier in the Recent Traumatic Episode Protocol (R-TEP). Newtown is an hour's drive from us and our first action was to find the EMDR clinicians in that area and call to offer our assistance. We located the therapists via personal contacts and by using the www.emdria.org website's "Find a Therapist" link.

Needs Assessment

Our TRN traveled to meet with the Newtown clinicians the next day, offered support, and conducted a needs assessment. The four Newtown EMDR clinicians were suffering their own losses from the shooting and anticipated being swamped in their practices in the weeks ahead. There were five immediate needs identified and met:

1. *Training in Recent Events EMDR Protocols and in Stabilization/Resourcing Protocols.* Restricted EMDR Protocols (R-TEP: Shapiro & Laub, 2007; A-TIP, Kiessling, personal communication) and grounding, calming, and self-control techniques (Shapiro, E. Four Elements Exercise for Stress Management) were reviewed along with Extended Resourcing Protocols (Korn & Leeds, 2002). Material sent from Robbie Adler-Tapia regarding mental health disaster response was also electronically provided for review. Engraved EWAF (Earth, Water, Air, Fire) bracelets with attached grounding, self-calming, and self-control instructions were placed in baskets with information about HAP and our TRN. Newtown clinicians distributed them to their own clients as well as to schools, hair salons, and diners so that the community could quickly learn a resource and so that they knew how to access treatment for first responders through our TRN.
2. *Emotional Support for Newtown Therapists in the Months Ahead.* Immediate pro bono EMDR treatment for therapists was offered and provided as a resource for their own trauma processing and resiliency building for the trying weeks and months ahead.
3. *EMDR Referrals for Area First Responders and Community Citizens.* We provided Newtown clinicians with a vetted list of EMDR therapists in the state of Connecticut (CT) by networking quickly with EMDR consultants throughout CT.
4. *Train CT Child EMDR Therapists in Disaster Response Protocols and the Group Treatment Protocol (Jarero, Artigas, & Hartung, 2006).* Carolyn Settle came from Arizona three weeks after the disaster to provide this training through HAP.
5. *Providing Self-Care.* Helping the clinicians feel that we supported their emotional well-being and bodily health was an essential part of our initial work and continued in the months ahead through pro bono massage certificates and a special spa day set up in a Sandy Hook office for the Newtown therapists.

Networking

Our next step was to network with Newtown and CT State first response organizations, schools, and non-EMDR clinicians to offer education about EMDR and our TRN services. In considering this particular massacre, we broadened our definition of First Responders from fire, police, EMDR, and mental health clinicians to include family members (children and adults directly impacted by the shooting), teachers, and clergy. In continuing our concern for area therapists, we held a workshop for Newtown and surrounding area therapists in grounding and stabilization techniques for children and adults, and introduced how EMDR could help in both an individual and group format, if and when requested.

EMDR Based Treatment and Training

As an outgrowth of our increasing connection with the Newtown clinicians, word began to spread about EMDR treatment effectiveness and our TRN expanded its membership. Our 12 clinicians traveled up to the Newtown area to provide up to three pro bono EMDR sessions to children, state troopers, police, clinicians, teachers, and parents, with referrals as needed. The Newtown Youth and Family Services agency requested training in EMDR, and HAP organized an EMDR Part 1 training. Our TRN offered one to three R-TEP sessions to enrolled trainee clinicians prior to their Part 1 Training of the EMDR Basic Training. This "Therapy for Newtown Therapists" project has proceeded very well. After the Part 1 training, the Newtown therapists reported that the R-TEP sessions helped to clear out some of their own trauma from the shooting in their community, excited them more about learning EMDR, and aided in their learning experience of EMDR therapy.

Healing the Healers

The idea to provide EMDR trainees with EMDR treatment prior to their training was borne out of a "Therapy for Therapists" project in New Orleans, coordinated by Sue

Evans, HAP volunteer, in New Orleans following Hurricanes Katrina and Rita. During HAP's ongoing efforts via Bob Gelbach to provide training and consultation to Gulf Coast clinicians, Katy Murray, Sue Evans, and I were asked by EMDR clinicians in New Orleans to create an EMDR treatment project for them and their Gulf Coast colleagues. They reported suffering from what we later came to identify as "shared traumatic reality" (Baum, 2010) and their small contingent of EMDR clinicians were too interconnected to provide treatment to each other. Intensive sessions were offered three times a week to the clinicians with the EMDR treatment target being Hurricane Katrina. While this treatment was provided 3 years after the hurricane, treatment results were significant and provided post-trauma symptom relief for the Gulf Coast clinicians (Alter-Reid et al., 2010). The implications of this project for intervention in disaster areas included the following important suggestions:

- Build resilience of clinicians through resourcing and treating trauma
- Identify and educate responders about shared traumatic realities
- Bring in clinicians from outside the community to treat the local therapists who also may have been primary trauma sufferers
- Provide EMDR treatment to clear out trauma before Part I training so that learning can be optimized rather than compromised by traumatic stress
- Model effective EMDR treatment by seasoned EMDR clinicians to optimize EMDR training and learning

The implications of this research project were put to use in Newtown. Along with treating trainees, we encourage our own TRN clinicians as first responders "in the field" to get their own EMDR treatment as they do and/or after doing the clinical work in Newtown with first responders (Marilyn Luber, personal communication, 2010).

Supporting the TRN Clinicians

Circles of support for our TRN clinicians came from EMDR therapists around the country, making our TRN's response truly feel like an EMDR community effort.

- Our community of HAP therapists from across the country gave of themselves: Provision of pro bono consultation and resources for our clinicians including immediate assistance from Carolyn Settle, Ana Gomez, Barbara Korzun, and Susan Schaefer.
- Sue Evans and Susan Schaefer from MN provided ongoing counsel and support to me on all levels of the mind and heart of our TRN work.
- Barbara Korzun and Robert Gelbach, former Executive Directors of HAP, shared lessons learned from past HAP disaster projects including Hurricane Katrina, the Columbine shooting, and the Indonesian tsunami.
- Carol Martin, current Executive Director of HAP, and Nancy Simons, Clinical Director, provided support.
- Robbie Adler-Tapia and Carolyn Settle from AZ provided ongoing consultation on disaster intervention and Beverly Chasse shared Arizona TRN's materials. Ana Gomez provided consultation for our child therapist.
- Karen Lansing from CA sent first responder materials for our TRN and trainees. Deany Laliotis provided wisdom for written materials sent to the State.
- Many HAP Trainers, Facilitators, and Consultants are readied to provide ongoing consultation to newly EMDR trained Newtown therapists.
  - In keeping with our commitment to healing the healers, our TRN considered the emotional and professional support that the HAP administrative staff deserved in the wake of responding to Hurricane Sandy and the Newtown shooting within three-months' time. We asked Dr. Ruth Heber from New York to provide this support and she became initiated as an official HAP volunteer that day. It's been quite an EMDR community effort!

Also, support came from other clinicians in the area. A group of Somatic Experiencing practitioners and Biodynamic Cranio-Sacral therapists offered us pro bono bodywork to help alleviate our compassion fatigue.

These circles of support have "held" us in "Winnicott-ian" fashion (Modell, 1976), enabling our TRN clinicians to continue offering training and treatment.

TRN Clinician Self-Care

Within our TRN, we supported each other in self-care efforts through ongoing peer support, consultation, and brief EMD treatment. The clinicians were contacted following their sessions to offer debriefing and reminders about self-care. This included encouraging needs assessments on how to keep balance in our lives, maintain boundaries, and not stretching beyond our own individual limits. During debriefing, if any of our clinicians reported distress or unprocessed images, thoughts, emotions, or sensations from their sessions, EMD or other restricted protocols were used to help them reprocess the memories. At TRN meetings, we reviewed and discussed the importance of buffering ourselves against vicarious trauma, compassion fatigue, and secondary PTSD. These are risk factors of working intensely with trauma victims (Figley, 2002; Pearlman & Maclan, 1995). This was especially important as we were trying to balance our private practices with travel to, and clinical work in, Newtown. Emphasis was given to taking care of our bodies with proper sleep, exercise, and nutrition and to spending time with family and friends. We made suggestions that responders do bodywork such as cranio-sacral therapy, massage therapy, and/or yoga, as body therapies are known ways to reduce stress. Additionally, we invited Millie Grenough, one of our EMDR local clinicians, to a meeting to teach us energetic discharge techniques for releasing our accumulating stress (Grenough, 2012). We plan to continue to do stress relief exercises at all our follow-up TRN meetings and remain accountable to each other by reporting on steps we are taking for self-care.

From the start, we emphasized the practice of self-care at educational workshops in Newtown where resourcing with butterfly hugs, breathwork (Kabat-Zinn, 2012), and pendulation techniques (Levine, 1997) were demonstrated and taught. During individual treatment, reminders were given at the close of R-TEP first responder sessions to therapists to reflect on their needs and listen to their bodies. Referrals were often made for exercise, bodywork, and mindfulness.

In heading up the efforts of the TRN's Healing the Wounded Healers, I often reflected on how members of our TRN kept making room for doing more clinical work with the primary sufferers of Newtown. It felt like there was something else going on; there seemed to be something innately healing from doing the work itself. As clinicians, bearing witness to the transformation from traumatic shock to healing during EMDR sessions was extraordinary. It felt as though the transmutation of experience/memory happening in our presence as clinicians was becoming encoded into our own neural networks by way of attunement and mirror neuron activity. These experiences may have increased our own adaptive memory networks of spiritual growth and transformation. Many of our clinicians felt they grew tremendously in their work and were becoming more effective EMDR clinicians in the few months since working in Newtown. While a bit disconcerting to think that we could grow and benefit in the midst of horror, I think we need to name, reflect, and embrace this as a side-effect of doing disaster work.

Here are some reflections on their clinical TRN work and on their self-care techniques.

Betty Rich, PhD:

It feels like an honor and privilege to be able to do this work. To be trusted to be able to help, and to know that I have the skills and experience to be worthy of that trust is incredibly powerful and satisfying at a personal and professional level. It feels like I'm supposed to be doing this work at this time in my life.

Having the connection to other experienced therapists who I can learn from, feeling supported in the work, and the intellectual challenge and professional growth from being with the group is tremendously satisfying. I feel nurtured and held by my colleagues, and know that I can call upon any of them if I need to debrief, or if I need help with procedural or logistical issues. I feel that my own experience and skills are valued by the group and it's exciting to be a part of such a quality team.

I have found it important to keep my schedule largely intact—seeing my existing patients, eating at the times I usually eat, exercising three times per week, getting enough sleep, etc. I have asked for extra TLC from home, for example, my husband cooks me nice dinners so I don't have to think about that when I'm working more than usual. I utilize the light bar in my office if I have imagery that I want to process; I just sit and let it run while mentally running through the things I've heard and seen that day.

I have noticed that at times during R-TEP processing when I'm tapping the hands of the client, I follow my hands with my eyes as well. This seems to help lower my own physiological arousal and keep me in my own window of effectiveness. I don't do this on every set, but I've noticed doing it from time to time, and find it interesting, wondering if anyone else does this. I also always take the deep breath between sets along with the clients, and have made this part of my EMDR practice for years. It both reminds them to do it and keeps us connected, helping with pacing. I protect myself from overload from media, watching enough TV news to keep current, but not overdoing it. I watch escapist type movies and comedies, Daily Show, etc. to be reminded of other parts of life. I say no to requests that exceed my existing coping abilities of the moment, and trust that others will be able to pick up the slack.

Valerie Gillies, LMFT:

For years, I maintained a small practice, working exclusively with children who have attachment and trauma issues. Once a month group consultation, peppered with outside support from masters when needed, kept me in a great space that I could not imagine leaving. My only concerns were about which delicious workshop or conference I could fit into my schedule next. A few days after the tragedy, I began treating a first responder and his family. Then, one by one, little ones appeared with parents, shaky and obviously not themselves. They needed me to be calm, centered, present, and playful. Self-care was not optional. But, it took nearly hitting a wall of exhaustion for me to realize that.

Some wise and experienced team members gently led me to see: (a) I cannot do it all, so I need to stick, firmly, to what I do best (children). Stretching to work with adults sucks the life out of me, so I fortified my will and referred them to others. (b) I need to embrace support, and get over any embarrassment about asking for help or making mistakes—yes, be content that my best is good enough. Many geographically distant EMDR therapists and the local Somatic Experiencing Practitioner community are treating, advising, and encouraging us. I connect daily with people on my team, and those in the larger circle of support, and am reminded that I am not in this alone. (c) I work physical release into client sessions. Deep breathing, shaking arms and legs to get the nasty feelings out, and playfully moving around help me and my clients center simultaneously. We are both in better shape at the end of sessions. (d) At home, I am using the strategies of a mother with small children, grabbing respite and rejuvenation whenever I can. No week goes by without bodywork, whether it is qigong, pedicure, or massage. My morning exercise time is sacred, as are my Epsom salt soaks before bed. I've had a few stolen overnights with my husband. If it feels good, I do it. If not, and it's not absolutely necessary, it's off my list. In an unlikely package, I was given the opportunity to open my world.

Dawn Roy, LCSW:

It has been two months since the tragic events of 12/14/12 Sandy Hook E.S. in Newtown, CT. I have been fortunate to be connected with the Fairfield County TRN that was immediately mobilized the day after this event. In the past two months, I have worked with four first responders, four mothers, and one father using the R-TEP protocol. In addition, I have worked closely with our team to deliver group presentations regarding Trauma and the use of EMDR. The individual work using R-TEP has resulted in a reported decrease of negative symptoms and an overall improvement of well-being. Clients have also been provided with stabilization and grounding exercises that they can utilize outside of the sessions.

It is to be expected that we, the helpers, would be impacted by the very work that we have done with clients (hearing the graphic details of the events and bearing witness to the intense pain and suffering of the clients who have experienced this). We have recognized that we have needed to process the intensity of this work and move it through our own brains and bodies. For many of us, the events of 12/14/12 have impacted our lives both personally and professionally. Doing our own work has been a critical piece to healing ourselves on both fronts: personally and professionally.

For me, regular consultation with my peers from the FCTRN, as well as somatic experiencing work with a provider, have been instrumental in my own healing. And then, of course, ongoing manicures and trips to the gym have also been excellent sources of self-care.

Michael Crouch, LCSW, Co-Coordinator, Fairfield County TRN:

Since the Christmas Day fire, I've watched my community of fellow EMDR therapists grow and found a network of colleagues who are dedicated to the work of healing those impacted by tragedy—therapists willing to give of their time and talents freely.

I've had the opportunity to get to know many of the first responders in our communities and am humbled by their courage and the compassion and caring they bring to their jobs. Whether it was the firemen in Stamford or the police in Newtown, all feel deeply for the victims of tragedies in their communities and go into battle with caring for others as their principal concern. It's been an honor to work with them.

Having the colleagues in the Trauma Recovery Network (TRN) to reach out to has been an invaluable resource for me in caring for myself. If I've had a question, struggled with what I've heard in a session, needed to talk about an EMDR protocol, or just needed support, I've had a network of friends/colleagues that I trust and respect to call. It's work we should not do alone. I did take a vacation to hug my grandsons and I will schedule an EMDR session to process through what we have heard and experienced secondhand.

Susan Marcus, LCSW:

In the aftermath of the Sandy Hook School shooting I treated two local area therapists in the "Therapy for Therapists" project and one Sandy Hook parent. Each of the three had very different responses to the tragedy. One had their own past trauma triggered, the second had a cultural trauma triggered, the third dealt more directly with the recent events. All processed strong emotions during their sessions.

Since I have family in Sandy Hook, working with these people was both deeply rewarding and challenging. I was acutely aware that had the events happened on any other day—Thursday, instead of that Friday—I could have been a mourner, rather than a helper. As a therapist, I was deeply moved by the process my clients went through, but later in the day or even the next day, I was sometimes hit with my own emotional response. I was very aware of how important self-care would be and that the excuse that I didn't have time was dangerous. And so I deliberately squeezed into my schedule having a massage, exercise, I made sure to get to a monthly women's group to which I belong, and I did some self-administered EMDR.

Other TRN members were: Ingeborg Haug, D.Min, LMFT; Linda Rost, LCSW; Libby Schreiber, LCSW; Jeanette Trujillo, PsyD; and Kate Wheeler, PhD.

Summary

We have learned many lessons from our TRN work in Newtown. Having a TRN in place in our own local community set the stage for more effective action in Newtown. Without it, we would have not have been able to respond as quickly. Being embraced by a national and international community of EMDR therapists, before even reaching out to them for resources, information, and expertise, was heartwarming and enhanced our work. Reaching beyond the EMDR community to offer EMDR treatment to the mental health community at large helped to stabilize and strengthen the therapists' capacity to provide therapy. We have discovered that the model that emerged from Hurricane Katrina has been used effectively with the Newtown disaster and can therefore have efficacy in future TRN applications. We look forward to collaborating with other TRN chapters across the country in sharing ideas, models, and blueprints for intervention following disasters, with particular emphasis on fortifying and healing the wounded healers.

Finally, at both the professional and personal levels, we learned that in the midst of horror, solid EMDR treatment can elicit the triumph of the human spirit. To be part of, and witness to, this transformation deepens all of us.

I wish to thank all the therapists who stepped up to provide pro bono work and consultation.

Note: More information about Cranio-sacral therapy can be found at www.craniosacral therapy.org

SUMMARY SHEET:
Community Trauma: A Blueprint for Support and Treatment for Trauma Recovery Network (TRN) Responders From the Newtown, CT, Tragedy

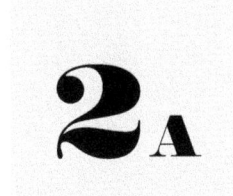

Karen Alter-Reid
SUMMARY SHEET BY MARILYN LUBER

Name: _____ Diagnosis: _____

☑ Check when task is completed, response has changed, or to indicate symptoms.

Note: This material is meant as a checklist for your response. Please keep in mind that it is only a reminder of different tasks that may or may not apply to your incident.

Introduction

Beginning a TRN   ☐ Completed

☐ Call EMDR colleagues
☐ Contact EMDR HAP for assistance in shaping goals
☐ Network with local fire and police departments
☐ Traumatology workshops
☐ EMDR education

First Responders also include:

☐ Mental Health Clinicians
☐ TRN Members

Preparation   ☐ Completed

☐ Understand "Shared Traumatic Reality"
☐ Caring for Our Own Therapists Chairperson Appointed

How to begin TRN response to nearby town with no TRN:

Locate therapists

☐ Personal Contact
☐ Find a Therapist Link (www.emdria.org)
☐ Other: _____
_____

Needs Assessment

1. Training in Recent Events EMDR Protocols and Stabilization/Resourcing Protocols
   - ☐ R-TEP
   - ☐ A-TIP
   - ☐ 4 Elements Exercise for Stress Management
   - ☐ Extended Resourcing Protocols
   - ☐ Mental Health Disaster Response Material
   - ☐ Create baskets for distribution in community with Four Elements Exercise instructions and information about HAP and TRN
   - ☐ Distribute baskets

2. Emotional Support for Therapists
   - ☐ Pro bono EMDR treatment for therapists offered

3. EMDR Referrals for Area First Responders and Community Citizens
   - ☐ Create vetted list of EMDR therapists in the state through networking with EMDR Consultants

4. Train Child EMDR Therapist in Disaster Response Protocols and the Group Treatment Protocol
   - ☐ Training in Child Disaster Response Protocols

Networking ☐ Completed

- ☐ First Response organizations
- ☐ Schools
- ☐ Non-EMDR clinicians—offer education about EMDR and TRN services

Broaden definition of First Responders to include: ___ firemen ___ policemen ___ EMDR and MH clinicians ___ family members directly impacted by event ___ teachers ___ clergy

For Therapists in the Area ☐ Completed

- ☐ Grounding and Stabilization Techniques for children and adults
- ☐ Introduction to EMDR in individual and group format

EMDR Based Treatment and Training ☐ Completed

- ☐ Pro bono EMDR treatment (1–3 sessions)
- ☐ Train therapists in EMDR
- ☐ Do 1-3 R-TEP sessions with enrolled trainee clinicians prior to Part 1 ☐ Completed

Healing the Healers (see above) ☐ Completed

- ☐ Teach resourcing and treat trauma to build therapist resilience
- ☐ Identify and educate responders about shared traumatic realities
- ☐ Bring in outside community clinicians to treat primary trauma sufferers
- ☐ Model effective EMDR treatment by seasoned EMDR clinicians to optimize EMDR training and learning

Supporting the TRN Clinicians ☐ Completed

- ☐ Seek support from HAP
- ☐ Seek support from the EMDR community
- ☐ Seek support from the bodywork community

TRN Clinician Self-Care

- ☐ Peer Support
- ☐ Consultation
- ☐ Brief EMD treatment
- ☐ Contact clinician after sessions:
    - ☐ To debrief as needed
        - ☐ Evaluate if EMD/other restricted protocols needed
    - ☐ To remind about self-care
        - ☐ Balance in lives
        - ☐ Maintain boundaries

TRN meetings include discussion of buffering against vicarious trauma, compassion fatigue, and secondary PTSD ☐ Completed

- ☐ Proper sleep
- ☐ Exercise
- ☐ Nutrition
- ☐ Spend time with family and friends
- ☐ Body work (cranio-sacral, massage, yoga, etc.)
- ☐ Doing stress relief exercises during the meeting
- ☐ Each member reports on self-care steps
- ☐ Teach self-care at educational workshops
    - ☐ Butterfly hug
    - ☐ Breath work
    - ☐ Pendulation techniques
- ☐ During individual treatment
    - ☐ Reminders to reflect on needs and listen to bodies
    - ☐ Referrals to self-care practitioners as needed

Self-Care Techniques Used by TRN Responders ☐ Completed

- ☐ Feeling valued in the group
- ☐ Keep schedule intact: eating, enough sleep, extra TLC
- ☐ Utilize the light bar in office and run through the things seen and heard that day
- ☐ When tapping, follow my own hands with my eyes
- ☐ Take a deep breath between sets with clients
- ☐ Cut down on too much media
- ☐ Enjoy escapist movies and comedies
- ☐ Say no to requests that exceed my coping abilities at the moment
- ☐ Trust others will pick up the slack
- ☐ Embrace support
- ☐ Ask for help
- ☐ Be content with doing the best I can do
- ☐ Get support from other EMDR therapists
- ☐ Connect daily with people on my team—I am not alone
- ☐ Use physical release in client sessions such as deep breathing, shaking arms and legs to get the nasty feelings out
- ☐ Grab respite and rejuvenation when I can
- ☐ Do body work such as qigong, pedicure, or massage
- ☐ Morning exercise
- ☐ Epsom salt baths
- ☐ Time with significant other
- ☐ If it is not necessary, it is off my list
- ☐ Go to monthly women's/men's group

We learned that in the midst of horror, solid EMDR treatment can elicit the triumph of the human spirit. To be part of, and witness to, this transformation deepens us all.

Vicarious Trauma and EMDR

3

Derek Farrell

Personal Reflection

My first visit to Asia occurred in the aftermath of the Turkish earthquake in 1999, an earthquake of such power and magnitude that it claimed the lives of over 45,000 people. This 7.6 Richter-scale natural disaster had at its epicenter the industrialized town of Izmit in northwest Turkey. As it occurred at 3 a.m., many of the town's residents were understandably in bed and had no chance of escape. The damage to Izmit itself was immense, as many of its buildings had not been designed or constructed to withstand earthquakes, certainly not earthquakes of this size. Whole districts were simply razed to the ground. Even Istanbul, Turkey's largest city, some 50 miles northwest, experienced destruction. The main highway between Istanbul and Turkey's capital, Ankara, buckled, resulting in multiple vehicle crashes. Since the initial earthquake on August 17, the region was subjected to frequent aftershocks that caused more destruction, more terror, more trauma, more casualties, more fatalities, and more survivors.

Two months after the earthquake, our minibus—travelling initially along the road from Istanbul to Izmit before turning toward Yalova—pulled up beside an isolated compound. This was a community of family homes built in an area of natural beauty. Since crossing into Asia, the damage that we were witnessing all around us was simply overwhelming. This was a sweeping, and seemingly endless, landscape of sheer destruction. George Orwell once stated that, *"An earthquake is such fun when it is over."* There did not seem much evidence of *"fun"* here, just simply devastation. What was Orwell thinking of? I was witnessing miles and miles of complete and utter wreckage, the likes of which I certainly had never witnessed before.

The day had begun in what seemed a lifetime away in Istanbul. For the past week, I had been facilitating, as part of an EMDR Humanitarian Assistance Program, EMDR training for Turkish mental health workers. After the training, many of the participants were returning to refugee camps to, hopefully, practice their newly acquired EMDR skills. Members of the team were asked if we would be willing to go to the camps to offer support and live EMDR clinical supervision to some of the training participants. This seemed such a wonderful opportunity, a truly unique experience to make a further contribution. This EMDR HAP training, one of the first of its kind, had gone so well. For me personally, it had been a profoundly enriching experience. But now, looking at this compound of carnage, the EMDR training felt like we had been working in nothing but an isolated cocoon on the other side of the world.

As the endless devastation of the Turkish landscape kept coming mile after mile, the atmosphere among the occupants within the minibus became more and more subdued.

Memories of laughter and of teaching our Turkish colleagues to sing the famous England rugby anthem of *"Swing Low, Sweet Chariot"* the night before seemed a somewhat distant memory, somehow now trivial and insignificant, seemingly incongruent. I was struggling to find words to try to make sense of what it was we were actually witnessing.

For days during the EMDR training, we had all heard countless tales of participants' personal experiences. But there is a huge difference between hearing it and witnessing it. This was, after all, the reality of natural disasters. The idea of visiting EMDR training participants, participants we had come to know and made connections with and were now back working in the refugee camps, seemed a good idea at the time. Here was a unique opportunity to provide live EMDR clinical supervision—an opportunity I grasped willingly. Understandably, the refugee camps where our Turkish EMDR training participants were now working were strategically placed so as to best help large populations of people. To get to these camps required witnessing firsthand the destructive potency and devastation of this powerful force of nature. *"It will be fine,"* I thought, *"I'm resilient, I'm strong."* After all, we are trauma therapists, *"Right?" "I can cope,"* my psychotherapy, previous trauma, and EMDR training would provide me with a shield of immunity. Sure it will be fine!

What stood before us was a deserted house or—to be more precise—only half of it as—remarkably—its right part was perfectly intact. It looked like a family home, a home I imagined to be full of memories and a rich abundance of lived experiences. The left side of the house looked like it had been simply ripped away. The place looked like it was on a Hollywood movie blockbuster set, and I expected, at any point, to hear *"Lights, camera, and action!"* But this was not Hollywood, this was western Turkey. This was not a disaster movie set, this was a real life disaster zone.

As we gazed at this quite incredible *"half-house,"* nobody in the party spoke. There was nothing to say. What could we say? What could I say? I found myself unable to even engage in eye contact with my fellow colleagues. Looking more closely at the house, I saw the remnants of a kitchen where on the table were all the plates and crockery from the night before, still in situ. By now, the remaining leftovers had disintegrated but it still highlighted a powerful vision of a social gathering, a family meal that had taken place just hours before the earthquake.

Since my arrival in Istanbul, I had witnessed firsthand the warmth and generosity of Turkish hospitality. I now felt hugely emotional and wanted to weep. Yet, at the same time, I could not communicate my distress to my fellow EMDR colleagues. Part of my vulnerability was feeling distressed about my being distressed in such a devastating environment thousands of miles from home. I didn't know what to say, how to feel, what to think, or how to be at that very moment in time. Looking at this kitchen table, now, in this half dwelling, I felt that I knew that people probably lost their lives here, right in this very spot, right in this very home.

At that moment, the UK felt as if it were light-years away in another part of the universe. Suddenly, I felt profoundly overwhelmed, overwhelmed by such a strong feeling of my own insignificance: *"Why had I accepted coming to Turkey so easily? How could I think that I could do even the slightest thing to make even the remotest bit of difference? Who was I kidding?"* I felt like a complete and utter fraud standing there. I pretended that some dust had gotten into my eye and throat to explain the sudden tears and my inability to find my voice. Thankfully, no one commented. It was too much to even contemplate how this must all be for them. I was grateful for the silence.

Our journey continued on to the refugee camp in Yalova. Upon entering the camp, I was struck by its sheer size. It was enormous, with seemingly thousands of people residing there. At its entrance, members of the Turkish military met us in readiness to show us around the camp. Even though I had known that this was going to happen, I now felt extremely uncomfortable about it. My sense was that this was akin to voyeurism and therefore my instinct was to decline. However, my English reserve felt that it would be impolite to refuse. We were shown tens and tens of rows of tents by the camp military commander, tents that were now the temporary homesteads of families, friends, and fellow members of their communities. As we were walking around, something struck me about many of the camp's residents; it was the clothes that many were wearing. These people looked like they were affluent and wealthy. I do not know why I found this more shocking. The camp commander confirmed that many of the camp's residents had simply lost everything: *"There is a lot of anger here, a lot of anger."* In naïive crassness, I remember asking him, *"Who were they angry with?"* and he told this story:

> In the aftermath of the Turkish earthquake, God and the Devil decided to call a truce and agreed to meet in Istanbul. In order to reinforce the truce, they decided to build a road between heaven and hell. When the Devil arrived back in hell, he rounded up all the road engineers, architects, and builders that he could find. True to his word, the Devil started the long arduous process of building the road from hell. After many, many months, the Devil had reached the halfway point, the location where the two roads were scheduled to meet as one. However, neither God, nor the road from heaven, was anywhere to be seen. So the Devil waited, and waited, but still no road arrived. The Devil, overwhelmed with fury, called out to God. "Why have you failed to meet your end of our bargain and build the road from heaven?" To which God replied, "I apologize; I had every intention of honoring our agreement. However after our last meeting, I returned to heaven and found that actually all the Turkish road builders, engineers, and architects were all in hell!"

The fact that so many of the people's houses had collapsed because of poor design and the use of poor quality materials played a significant part in why the death toll in western Turkey was as high as it was.

We were then taken to another part in the center of the camp where there was a queue of people patiently waiting in a line. The refugee camp was expecting a United Nations delivery of mattresses. In the front of the line was a man wearing a very smart suit and overcoat. As he stood in silence, there seemed a certain dignity about him, yet at the same time, he seemed disconnected to all that was going on around him. He certainly seemed oblivious to my observing him. At that moment, the UN truck arrived, however, it did not stop at its allocated place, and instead it went some 50 meters farther up the road. As a consequence, what was at first an orderly queue now turned into a mad scramble for the new, rapidly off-loaded mattresses being bundled out of the truck. This man suddenly became very angry and acutely distressed and started to shout at his fellow incumbents, but he was simply ignored by all around him. A soldier informed me that the man was just angry because he had been waiting in this queue for four hours to ensure that he got a mattress for his family. *"It happens all the time,"* he said. This man's distress was palpable. I felt helpless. I so much wanted to give him my mattress.

That evening, on our return to Istanbul, in order to thank the EMDR HAP team, we had been invited to an evening cruise on a private boat sailing the river Bosporus. The whole experience of this HAP training had been incredible. There were so many wonderful memories of the training, facilitating, and working alongside fellow EMDR international colleagues, the hospitality of the Turkish people, the fun, the humor, the singing, the laughter, and the dancing. Listening to EMDR participants' experiences during the practicums had been a privilege; hearing about their pain, their loss, and how their lives had been inextricably changed as a result of the earthquake, the aftershocks, and their subsequent legacy. Although the spirit within the group was seemingly very high, I was aware of feeling very distracted while on board. I caught sight of a label on a bottle of red wine that the waiters were serving members of the EMDR HAP training team. I recognized this label and knew it to be an expensive wine. As a result, I could not drink it. I felt guilty. How could I drink such expensive wine when people were suffering still in the aftermath of the earthquake? I could not wait to get off the boat. I just wanted to go home.

Returning back to work in the United Kingdom after my experiences in Turkey was hugely difficult. I was very quiet and not really interacting much with my fellow National Health Service (NHS) work colleagues. It felt like my emotions were all over the place and I found myself being unusually argumentative during team meetings. Work was a busy psychology department and none of my colleagues seemed remotely interested in the Turkish EMDR HAP training experience. The only comment I received came from my Head of Department who had asked me if I had had a good time. *"Had a good time? Are you for f**king real? It's a f**king disaster zone,"* I shouted! He reprimanded me severely for swearing at him and threatened disciplinary action if I ever spoke to him like that again. It was the first and only time I had ever spoken like that to a manager in my entire professional career. He never forgave me despite my apologizing.

My way of surviving was to place all of my energy into maintaining quality in my clinical work with clients. However, I was finding it both cognitively and emotionally incredibly exhausting to keep going. It was taking all my energy to concentrate, which meant that I was having less and less energy for my home life. Over and over in my mind, I kept seeing images of the kitchen table and of the man's face waiting in line. I was starting to seriously doubt myself as a psychologist/psychotherapist. My clinical caseload consisted of a whole series of extremely difficult and complex trauma clients.

As time went by, I was increasingly feeling more isolated and unsupported. My clinical supervisor showed no real commitment toward either supporting or challenging me. On reflection, she seemed completely oblivious and disinterested in what was really going on. I had the sense to know that I was not OK, but I also felt ashamed to admit it. My situation was compounded by working in an environment with people who also seemed disconnected and disinterested. It is very hard to do good quality clinical work with trauma populations when you yourself are experiencing parallel trauma symptoms in an environment not really conducive to ensuring safety, support, self-preservation, and healing.

On reflection, when I look back at things now in terms of how I was functioning both personally and professionally at the time immediately post Turkey, the following symptoms were very much in evidence:

- Intrusive recollections—flashbacks, bad dreams, nightmares
- Clinical judgment and decision making was impaired
- Profound feelings of over-responsibility particularly with some of my complex trauma clients
- Overworking in clinical sessions with clients
- Significant imbalance between work and personal life
- Excessive hours of working both at the National Health Service (NHS) and private practice
- Trying to be more active in controlling other people's lives
- Emotional regulation was difficult
- Diminution in confidence and self-esteem
- Quality of personal relationships deteriorated
- Sense of disconnection
- Frequent headaches and migraines
- Loss of meaning, hope, and purpose
- Blame others instead of seeking understanding and productive collaboration
- Increased sensitivity to violence and trauma

In considering this list, each symptom seemed extremely distinct, however, many of these symptoms were profoundly subtle. A huge amount of my energy at the time was spent giving an outward appearance that there was absolutely nothing wrong at all. Remarkably, I never even remotely considered using EMDR or seeking any form of help and assistance with any of this.

Vicarious Trauma

My symptoms, mentioned above, are indicative of what Pearlman and Saakvitne (1995) call vicarious trauma. They determined that vicarious trauma creates a permanent transformation of a therapist's inner experience. They purport that the effects of vicarious trauma can be very significant although they acknowledge that symptoms are unique to the individual. They outline five attributes of vicarious trauma:

1. Alterations in self-identity and perception
2. Alterations in a person's sense of spirituality
3. Alterations in personal beliefs and assumptions
4. Physical and psychological symptoms
5. Impact upon interpersonal relationships

To explore these five attributes in more detail, Lansen and Haans (2004), Palm Polusny, and Follete (2004), and Pearlman (1995) consider that many of the symptoms of vicarious trauma listed below parallel the criteria of Post-Traumatic Stress Disorder (PTSD):

- Showing symptoms of post-traumatic stress disorder: nightmares, sleeplessness, intrusions, avoidance behavior, irritability
- Denial of client's trauma
- Overidentification with client
- No time and energy for oneself
- Feelings of great vulnerability
- Insignificant daily events are experienced as threatening
- Feelings of alienation
- Social withdrawal
- Disconnection from loved ones
- Loss of confidence that good is still possible in the world
- Generalized despair and hopelessness
- Loss of feeling secure
- Increased sensitivity to violence
- Cynicism
- Feeling disillusioned by humanity
- Disrupted frame of reference
- Changes in identity, worldview, spirituality
- Diminished self-capacities
- Impaired ego resources
- Alterations in sensory experiences

In order to be effective as psychotherapists in our work with clients requires, among many things, positive energy in maintaining an empathic connection between ourselves and our clients. It could be argued that vicarious trauma is an experience in which there is a loss of this positive energy. McCann and Pearlmann (1990) consider that vicarious trauma is often viewed as an indication of weakness on the part of the therapist and therefore implies that somebody is to blame. If effective psychotherapy involves empathic connection in deepening our understanding of humanity then vicarious trauma, they argue, is an occupational hazard. The vicarious trauma phenomenon provides a window of opportunity for healing, post-trauma growth, and personal and professional development.

As mentioned previously, I knew that post-Turkey 1999, I was not OK. Nonetheless, it took many months before I eventually sought help and assistance. What triggered it was my experiencing a dissociative episode. I recall sitting in my office early one morning at work staring at an Islamic prayer mat that I had bought in Turkey and had placed on a wall by my desk. The next thing I remember was hearing a knock on the door. It was my colleague asking if I wanted to go for lunch. When I looked at my watch, four hours had gone by. I was completely shocked and badly shaken by this experience. Where had those four hours gone? Nothing like this had ever happened to me before. It was time to seek help. Putting myself through psychotherapy, which included EMDR, to address my vicarious trauma was one of the hardest and best decisions I made.

EMDR, Narratives, and Vicarious Trauma

The outcome of psychotherapy proved to have a very powerful impact on me both personally and professionally. A great many changes came about as a consequence of this work and journey. Probably the most important healing aspect, initially, was in experiencing a profound reality check that what I was undergoing was actually understandable and was already known about in academic literature. At the time, I remember feeling greatly reassured by recalling the words of my therapist who had calmly stated, *"OK, so we now know what the problem is. It's important that you hold on to the fact that it is sortable."*

Although it is many years now since I completed this psychotherapy journey in relation to my vicarious trauma, I frequently reflect upon the help that I received, consider what I learned from the process, and evaluate how this has translated into my own clinical practice and how I now work with clients and therapists who experience vicarious trauma. As my understanding of vicarious trauma has deepened, I have found myself considering the wider perspectives of the multitude of narratives that exist within vicarious trauma. The psychotherapy I received was an integration of a number of psychotherapeutic approaches that included EMDR. In relation to the EMDR treatment, my therapist targeted, as would be expected, significant experiences that were causing presently held levels of distress. For example, the kitchen table, the man waiting in the queue, the incident with my head of department, etc. These were all targeted with productive outcomes. However, these were just a part of the narrative.

As my knowledge, understanding, and clinical application of EMDR has developed, to the point that I am now an EMDR Europe Accredited Trainer, reflecting upon my own experience of EMDR as a client has been immensely helpful. A product of this endeavor brings me back to this aspect of considering the multiple narratives that seem to me to be in evidence in our vicarious trauma client group. As a consequence, I would propose that there are in fact eight different narratives to consider in relation to an EMDR/Adaptive Information Processing (AIP) Case Formulation and Target Treatment Sequencing Plan. The rationale for considering eight narratives is that, in my experience of treating a great many clients and therapists with vicarious trauma, I am of the viewpoint that vicarious trauma never occurs in a vacuum. The trigger or catalyst is often the *"straw that broke the camel's back."* These multiple narratives include the following that are highlighted in Table 3.1.

Considering vicarious trauma from each of these narrative perspectives potentially enables the EMDR therapist to obtain a broader understanding of a client's symptoms and experiences. These multiple narratives have implications for the EMDR Phases of History Taking, Preparation, and Target Sequencing. For Phase 1: History Taking, it is important to ensure the following:

- All necessary background information is obtained from the client
- The Adaptive Information Processing (AIP) perspective when doing case conceptualization is considered in addition to utilizing diagnostic and case formulations
- The client meets the criteria of appropriateness for EMDR treatment
- Positive resources and stabilization/anchor points identified, so as to then develop an effective EMDR treatment target sequence plan.

Note: In the absence of positive resources and functioning anchor points, the client potentially may require more time spent, by the EMDR clinician, in the Preparation Phase of EMDR so as to maximize support and stabilization for the client.

Table 3.1 Multiple Narratives Within Vicarious Trauma

Narrative 1.	The narrative of *the story* itself
Narrative 2.	The *narrator*—who is telling the story
Narrative 3.	The narration—how the story is being told in terms of *affect*
Narrative 4.	The narrative *medium*—what methods are used to relate the narration
Narrative 5.	Co-narratives—narratives from the *perspectives* of significant others
Narrative 6.	Parallel narratives—what *other narratives* are going on concurrently
Narrative 7.	The narrative *"Here and Now"* or *"Time and Place"*—why is this story being told at this particular point in time and place?
Narrative 8.	The *narrative transaction*—how the narrative is heard by the listener from the view of the recipient

The Eight Multiple Narratives Within Vicarious Trauma

Narrative 1: The Narrative of the Story Itself

The client's story is important but this is just one part of the narrative. Sometimes the client's narrative may appear chaotic and lack structure; however the narrative emerges and unfolds over a period of time. Clients seldom provide their narratives in a clear, articulate, and chronological sequence.

Example: A Traffic Police Officer recounted a story of an incident for which he was in attendance that involved a road traffic collision between two vehicles where he was first on the scene. A car carrying a family of mother, father, and two young children was hit by another vehicle being driven by a young man who was severely intoxicated. The officer recalled the young man surviving the incident with only minor grazes but the family were horrifically injured with one of the children being declared dead at the scene. In eighteen years' service, he admitted that he had witnessed hundreds of horrific road traffic collisions, however the dichotomy of seeing paramedics trying to resuscitate this child and then seeing the young man unscathed, seemingly oblivious to all that was going on around him, stirred a powerful surge of anger within him. He described the feelings he had toward this young man as *"primitive, Neanderthal, and homicidal,"* declaring that, *"I remember clearly thinking that a custodial sentence was just not enough for people like him. I start to fantasize about what I could do to seriously hurt him, and make him realize what he'd done. Then I caught sight of myself. I was shocked that I was starting to think this way. That's when I knew I needed to see somebody."*

Narrative 2: The Narrator—Who Is Telling the Story

Narrative 2 considers the person behind the narrative: How are they choosing to tell their story, what methods are they using to convey their vicarious trauma, and why are they telling this narrative now? This will provide some clues around the balance between, first, EMDR target identification and selection and, second resource building and stabilization.

Example: In Narrative 1, we heard about a very experienced traffic police officer who had witnessed hundreds of serious road traffic collisions but admitted that he had *"never lost a night's sleep over them."* But, in having a more enhanced understanding of the story, it is important that we understand more about the story's narrator. What is it about this incident that makes it so different, so unique? Why does this incident stand out from simply hundreds of other road traffic collisions? The Police Officer stated that it was the *"dichotomy of seeing paramedics trying to resuscitate this child and then seeing the young man unscathed, seemingly oblivious to all that was going on around him, stirred a powerful surge of anger within him."* From an EMDR perspective, we would use this insight to assist the Police Officer in floating back to the earliest time that he felt that way using either previous incidents, negative cognitions, or an affect bridge.

Narrative 3: The Narration—How the Story Is Being Told in Terms of Affect

Clients struggling with Narrative 3 may require more time in preparation, stabilization, and resource building, for example, before proceeding toward desensitization and reprocessing of their vicarious trauma target material.

Example: A neonatal nurse sought psychological help following the death of a four-week-old baby who was born prematurely. She was a nurse with over 10 years' experience in the field. However, she could not talk about this incident without bursting into tears and crying uncontrollably. Her emotions felt chaotic which in turn frightened her further as she admitted to being fractious, vulnerable, raw, and fragmented. This manifested itself in huge surges of panic that, at times, completely overwhelmed her. She said, *"I just don't understand why I can't get a handle on my emotions, I just feel all over the place. I just feel so stupid and silly that this one incident is affecting my life in this way."*

Note: Etherington (2009) highlights that silence, as an entity, is also a narrative where words cannot penetrate. This silence can often reveal much about a client's affect. What is not said and spoken can often speak and reveal so much.

Narrative 4: The Narrative Medium—What Methods Are Used to Relate the Narration

Narrative 4 considers the medium in which clients feel more comfortable telling their story. In cases of shame or profound guilt, verbalizing the narrative might be too difficult and therefore Blore's EMDR *"Blind to Therapist Protocol"* may be a helpful tool for EMDR clinicians to consider. I have also had some vicarious trauma clients to whom asking to *"narrate the story verbally"* was rather akin to asking them to walk to the moon.

Example: One client, a prison officer who struggled with this aspect, debated the merits of writing it down, e-mailing it, posting it, drawing it, yelling it, and recording it. He thought about speaking to me on the phone, while in my office, while at home, at work, walking the dog, in a coffee shop, and yet still he could not move forward with it. What eventually worked was when I said to him, *"Come on, let's go for a walk."* Two minutes into the walk he opened up. It was the first time he had been able to talk about a really serious hostage situation he had witnessed at his place of work, a high security prison. At a critical, point he had frozen and later interpreted his response with a profound sense of shame and anguish. His symptoms were compounded by the ridicule and subsequent bullying he received from his colleagues, post incident. It transpired that this incident, as powerful as it was, was just one of a whole catalogue of events that highlighted serious flaws in the way in which the institution was being operated and managed.

Narrative 5: Co-Narratives—Narratives From the Perspectives of Significant Others

In understanding the wider and systemic aspects of vicarious trauma, Narrative 5 involves obtaining an understanding, where possible, from the narrator's significant others: wife, husband, partner, parent, family member, and so on. The reason why this is important is that it can often provide a vital, and broader, context to the client's vicarious trauma.

Example: A camera operator from a large news corporation came to see me, rather reluctantly, following a report that he had recently filmed about childhood atrocities in Africa with children being murdered as a consequence of witchcraft. He attended the session with his partner. Throughout the interview the partner did not say very much. The client presented a narrative that indicated that he was *"fine,"* *"did not need any help,"* *"time will sort it out."* His partner then prompted him to tell me about the incident that happened in Libya when he was filming a site in a civilian area that had just been hit by NATO missiles. He caught sight of the body of a young child, killed by the bomb blast, being cradled in his grief-stricken father's arms. At this point, the client started to cry inconsolably. The partner stated that the client had been a *"complete nightmare to live with"* post Libya, highlighting that he was always irritable, restless, and difficult to be with. "We are trying for a baby," she said. *"It's not been easy."* The client looked aghast. It was like there was a dawning of realization for him. This was the wake-up call and reality check that he needed.

Narrative 6: Parallel Narratives—What Other Narratives Are Going on Concurrently?

Narrative 6 considers the parallel narratives often running alongside the vicarious trauma incident.

Example: For the prison officer, it was important to know that his father, with whom he was extremely close, had suddenly died. For the camera operator it was the fact that he was facing the possibility of either losing his job, going freelance due to relocation of a large part of the organization in which he worked to another part of the UK, or of trying to become a father for the very first time. These provide vital insights into why potential multiple targets become important factors to be considered when selecting appropriate targets for EMDR processing.

Narrative 7: The Narrative "Here and Now" or "Time and Place"—Why Is This Story Being Told at This Particular Point in Time and Place?

Narrative 7 considers factors that may be in evidence in relation to why the story is being told *now*.

Example: To provide a larger context from my own situation, at the time of my own vicarious trauma in relation to the Turkish earthquake, I was in the middle of my PhD research exploring survivors' experiences of sexual abuse perpetrated by clergy. This research involved in-depth interviews with survivors about their sexual abuse experiences mainly perpetrated by Roman Catholic Priests, although the study did focus on other Christian denominations as well. The abuse survivors portrayed profoundly graphic narratives of sexual violence, emotional and psychological abuse, theological and spiritual distress, mental anguish, and trauma. Another important reality check was that I had hired a professional transcription secretary to type out all of the research interviews that I'd conducted. One day into the job, the secretary rang me as she was in an extremely distressed state. She informed me that she could not do the transcriptions as she had simply found it far too upsetting. I'm guessing that something must have been activated for her but it felt inappropriate to pursue this with her. This was not after all a psychotherapeutic relationship but a business transaction. However, I felt responsible for vicariously traumatizing her as a result of my PhD research. As a primary investigator of a research project, I found myself asking, *"What was my duty of care to this secretary?"* Later, when I went to her home to collect the tapes, she must have seen my car pulling up. She ran out of the house, thrust the box of tapes in my arms, and promptly went back in. She never said a word or looked at me. Several weeks later she e-mailed me to apologize and stated that she had found the survivors' stories just *"too overwhelming."* Distinctions about what you are responsible for and what not are important to consider. I came to realize that I was not responsible for the issue that got triggered for this secretary; however, I was responsible for not sufficiently preparing her about the depth and trauma content of the research interviews. My own disconnection from the material had, unwittingly, vicariously exposed this secretary to trauma. I have never forgotten this opportunity for learning in any subsequent research that I have been engaged in to date.

In addition, I was also facing anger from some members of the Roman Catholic Church hierarchy who were hostile to the research being undertaken in the first place. Even though my research focused on Christian denominations as a whole, criticism came only from members of the Roman Catholic faith. So, on one hand, I was hearing these incredibly powerful testimonies from clergy abuse survivors, many of whom were telling their story for the first time, and then, on the other, hearing ultra-defensive arguments from clerics and non-clerics questioning, *"Why are you doing this research?"* and accusing me of being *"anti-Catholic,"* and labeling me: *"It's people like you that are causing huge damage to the Roman Catholic Church."*

These were all powerful triggers that seemed to have a sort of constellation effect; however, it was the dissociative episode that acted as the most significant trigger for me to eventually seek out psychological help and support. Although the intrusive trauma symptoms were about Turkey, the wider context related to my clinical working environment, and my on-going PhD research into clergy sexual abuse. This was the point where I decided that it was *"time to heal."* I didn't want it to be getting in the way of my life any more. My therapist once asked me, *"What is the best bit about being you?"* I instantly answered, *"Being a Dad."*

This became a powerful means of stabilization and anchor point, a resource that I had never articulated in this way before. "Being a Dad" continues to be the most important aspect in my life by a considerable country mile.

Narrative 8: The Narrative Transaction—How the Narrative Is Heard by the Listener From the View of the Recipient

Narrative 8 is about how the client perceives his/her words are heard by the therapist.

Example: Several years after finishing therapy, I made contact with my therapist and asked if I could make an appointment to see her. In my e-mail to her I had written, *"I don't know if you would remember me but ....?"* When she replied, she commented on this point, asking, *"What on earth makes you think that I would not have remembered you?"* My fantasy was that at the end of our work together, she would have just moved on to the next client. My reason for contacting her was that I wanted to tell that I had been awarded my PhD. She was delighted. However, the session also acted as a form of debrief about our psychotherapeutic work together. She asked me, *"What it was about our work that you found helpful?"* This was a hard question for me to answer, as there were actually so many aspects. But one of the things I remember she provided me with was an important *reality check* when she fed back how she had heard my narrative. Her version of my narrative gave me a vital perspective that what I was in fact experiencing was valid, significant, important, and needed the uttermost attention *now*.

However, it is also essential, from the perspective of therapists' self-care, to be mindful of the potential susceptibility for vicarious trauma. Skovholt (2001) aptly compared the well-functioning psychotherapist to that of a healthy and vibrant tree. His analogy suggests that just as a tree must take in sunlight, water, and carbon dioxide to be strong enough to withstand the internal and external stressors of living, so too must psychotherapists work hard in relation to their own physical and psychological well-being. What keeps psychotherapists healthy and well-functioning are the vibrant branches of professional and personal activities, the nurturing soil of professional and personal relationships, and the deep roots of professional and personal ideology. My therapist disclosed that I had not been easy to work with because many of the issues I struggled with resonated with many of hers. Understandably, I did not know that at the time. One of the most humbling things she said to me was the following, *"Seeing how fragile and vulnerable you were really made me think about myself in that I came to recognize that it was important for me to be strong and solid for you. I had to take care of me, to take care of you. You taught me that. That's what I did. Why on earth did you think that I would not remember you?"*

Considering each of the narratives in these eight ways enables the EMDR clinician to be more mindful for the potential multiple layers involved in the client's overall story. The corollary of these multiple narratives may require the EMDR clinician to utilize a variety of different skills and interventions, including more resource building, stabilization techniques, and a target sequencing plan, in order to best meet the individual needs of the client, whether the EMDR clinician is working to a comprehensive treatment plan or symptom reduction. Although most of the narratives center on the client and significant others, the EMDR clinician is also important to consider within the context of the overall narrative. As the EMDR clinician is an agent of change in the psychotherapeutic process, then his/her narrative is a potential vulnerability for vicarious trauma, and, therefore, as such, needs to be protected, suitably resourced, and potentially mitigated for.

Reflecting on the outcome of therapy regarding my own vicarious trauma, there were a great many salient aspects that effectively contributed to a successful outcome from treatment. As I mentioned earlier, I came to recognize that I could not do this on my own. One of the consequences of this was that I needed to seriously consider my internal and external resources before coming to the conclusion that I needed to access more effective and productive ones, including a root and branch review of my personal, professional, and spiritual life. Table 2 contains a number of aspects that I considered helpful in relation to psychotherapists working with clients experiencing vicarious trauma.

Table 3.2 Action Points to Consider in Relation to Addressing Vicarious Trauma

1. Obtain, or utilize existing, good quality and effective clinical supervision and/or EMDR psychotherapy while at the same time being clear about the distinction and rationale for both
2. Be open and honest with yourself in acknowledging the difficulties you may be experiencing
3. Be open to listening to constructive feedback from clinical supervisors, managers, colleagues, friends, family, and loved ones, being mindful to hear the positives as well as any potential negatives
4. Perform the simple things well in taking care of yourself, maintaining a healthy diet, regular exercise, and generally making time for yourself
5. Undertake a complete review of your current client caseload, clinical supervision/consultation commitments, teaching and learning workload, extra curricula activity, etc.
6. Revisit *"old comforts,"* such as re-reading your favorite book, watching your favorite films or television series, visiting your favorite restaurants, listening to music you have not heard for a while
7. Give some critical consideration to issues such as work-life balance
8. Consider new opportunities for potential inclusion into your life, of a new hobby, or the vacation you always wanted to go on, and/or new friendships, etc.
9. Ask yourself about what really is *"important"* in your life, what are the areas of *"real"* priority?
10. *"Practice what you preach"*—play back the way in which you assist a client with vicarious trauma and ask yourself should their *"treatment"* be your *"treatment?"*
11. Keep a reflective journal, remembering that the benefits of it are not just for your clients, they can be yours also
12. Find physical places and people you can spend some *"quality time"* with and *"make it happen"*
13. Reintroduce yourself and reconnect with social networks and friends
14. Practice saying, *"No,"* and then feeling *"OK"* about it
15. Give yourself permission to allow somebody else to take care of you even if it is just for a while

Multiple Narratives and the EMDR Targeting Sequence Plan

If we consider each of the eight narratives involving the traffic police officer, the neonatal nurse, the prison officer, and the camera operator, one of the factors that they each had in common was that the trigger for seeking psychological assistance related to an occupational related incident perpetrated during the course of their professional duties and responsibilities. These triggers, albeit significant, needed to be considered within the context of each client's overall target sequence plan, past, present and future. Each of these experiences created presently held levels of distress because they were in some way connected with previous experiences where the information from these experiences had not been sufficiently processed and integrated into narrative memory. This presently held level of disturbance prepetuates vulnerability sufficient enough to influence future levels of functioning, interactions and performance. In essence this is the core component of the EMDR Adaptive Information Processing model, which considers the relationship between the past, present and future in relation to information processing.

In developing an effective EMDR Targeting Sequence Plan, a root and branch review of the client's personal and spiritual life needs to be carried out as well as all professional aspects relating to the client. What is often fascinating to consider in relation to spiritual and even existential trauma targets is that they may relate to aspects that are about the future in their orientation. Just as a narrative has a beginning, middle and end—but not necessarily in that order—this also parallels the EMDR AIP model in relation to Targeting Sequence planning regarding the past, present and future. Even though the goal is to acquire a comprehensive history from clients, EMDR therapists need to be cognizant that history taking is often a live and ongoing process and therefore the EMDR Target Sequence Plan will also be an evolving process.

In relation to vicarious trauma, Table 2 highlights a number of salient factors for EMDR psychotherapists to consider in both obtaining a comprehensive history and then to develop an effective EMDR Targeting Sequence Plan. For EMDR therapy to be effective requires self-care on behalf of the EMDR psychotherapist. These 15 points not only highlight aspects to consider in relation to EMDR psychotherapists own self-care but may also be used to identify their own EMDR Targeting Sequence Plan that could then be used for working through the vicarious target experiences.

Addressing Vicarious Trauma After EMDR HAP Projects

The EMDR HAP training in Turkey 1999 played a significant part in developing EMDR. As a team, we have much to be proud of in what we achieved. Today, Turkey is a very important, and flourishing, member of EMDR Europe. After the training, we each went our separate ways on the assumption that everybody was *"OK."* Addressing my own vicarious trauma did not make me more predisposed to further vulnerability in humanitarian work; in fact, it had the exact opposite effect. It provided me with greater resilience.

Post-Turkey, I feel profoundly honored to be involved in many EMDR humanitarian projects throughout the world in India, Palestine, Northern Ireland, Poland, and Thailand. Since 2007, other colleagues and I have been involved in an on-going EMDR HAP Europe project in Pakistan and have trained over 120 mental health workers in EMDR.

After the EMDR HAP training in Turkey, with the benefit of hindsight, a suggestion would be that there should have been an opportunity for the whole team to come together and disentangle the positives and negatives from the EMDR training experience. Within any EMDR humanitarian project, I think it is important that a member of the team is identified for assuming responsibility for providing psychological well-being support for team members. This pastoral support may never be called upon, but it should at least be explicitly available as a resource and as a means of normalizing the occurrence of vicarious trauma. In addition, the following, *EMDR Positive "Stay & Go" Scripted Protocol* should also be given due consideration. It contains five stages within a group exercise format that includes the following:

1. Being part of the EMDR training team
2. Acknowledging your contribution to one individual
3. Valuing yourself
4. Focusing on your needs as an individual
5. Grounding exercise—Group Share

EMDR Positive "Stay and Go" Group Exercise Scripted Protocol

1. Support of the Team

An individual is identified from within the EMDR HAP training team who assumes responsibility for psychological well-being support for the entire team.

2. Team Meeting

A team meeting is arranged at the end of the training to carry out the EMDR Positive "Stay & Go" Group Exercise to determine what positives from the training need to stay behind and what positives can be taken away.

3. EMDR Positive "Stay & Go" Group Exercise

Do the EMDR Positive "Stay & Go" Group Exercise with the entire EMDR HAP team.

First Stage—Being Part of the EMDR Training Team

Say, "*Just take a moment to ground yourself in this present space here as part of the EMDR HAP team.*"

_____
_____

Say, "*Mentally float-back over this EMDR HAP training and consider what contribution you have made to the team in being part of this EMDR HAP training experience.*"

_____
_____

Say, "*When you think about this contribution, identify a positive cognition (PC) connected to what this contribution says about you as an individual, right at this moment in time.*"

_____
_____

Say, "*Mindful of this positive cognition, feel and remember how your body experiences this positive cognition.*"

_____
_____

Say, "*Holding this positive contribution, your PC, and positive body sensation together, reinforce this important information by using slow bilateral stimulation such as the Butterfly Hug or any other bilateral stimulation to enhance this positive resource.*"

_____
_____

Say, "*Make a mental photograph of this resource.*"

_____
_____

Say, "*Ask yourself the question about this resource, 'Do I want this resource to stay here or do I want to take it away with me?'*"

_____
_____

Say, "*Respecting whatever decision you make, use any slow BLS or the Butterfly Hug to reinforce this.*"

_____
_____

Say, "Float-back over the entire training, then identify for yourself something positive that symbolizes being part of this EMDR HAP team."

Second Stage—Acknowledging Your Contribution to One Individual

Say, "Mentally float-back over the entire EMDR HAP training and consider what contribution you have made to just one individual that is part of this training experience. It could be as a participant, colleague, organizer, and so on."

Say, "When you think about this contribution, identify a positive cognition connected to what this contribution says about you as an individual—right at this moment in time."

Say, "Mindful of this positive cognition, feel and remember how your body experiences this positive cognition."

Say, "Holding your positive contribution to this individual in mind, with your positive cognition and positive body sensation, reinforce this by using any slow BLS or the Butterfly Hug to enhance this positive resource."

Say, "Make a mental photograph of this resource."

Say, "Then ask yourself the following question about this resource, 'Do I want this resource to stay here or do I want to take it away with me?'"

Say, "Respecting whatever decision you choose, use any slow BLS or the Butterfly Hug to reinforce this."

Third Stage—Valuing Yourself

Say, *"Mentally float-back over this entire EMDR HAP training and consider what you have learned most about yourself from this training experience."*

_____
_____

Say, *"When you think about this contribution, identify a positive cognition connected to what this contribution says about you as an individual right at this moment in time."*

_____
_____

Say, *"Mindful of this positive cognition, feel and remember how your body experiences this positive cognition."*

_____
_____

Say, *"Holding your positive contribution to yourself in mind, with your positive cognition and positive body sensation, reinforce this by using any slow BLS or the Butterfly Hug to enhance this positive resource."*

_____
_____

Say, *"Make a mental photograph of this resource."*

_____
_____

Say, *"Then ask yourself the following question about this resource, 'Do I want this resource to stay here or do I want to take it away with me?'"*

_____
_____

Say, *"Respecting whatever decision you choose, use any slow BLS or the Butterfly Hug to reinforce this."*

_____
_____

Fourth Stage: Focusing on Your Needs as an Individual

Say, *"Mentally float-back over this entire EMDR HAP training and consider what negatives you may be holding about this EMDR HAP training experience."*

_____
_____

Say, "Notice how your body responds when this memory is activated."

Say, "Take a moment to consider your choices about this target(s) and consider the following questions."

Say, "Then, ask yourself the following question about this issue(s): 'Do I want this target experience to stay here or do I want to take it away with me?'"

Say, "Is this a target(s) that needs to stay or go?"

Say, "If it needs to remain here, then would the Daniel's Self-Care for EMDR Practitioners be sufficient?"

If it is helpful to do Daniel's Self-Care for EMDR Practitioners, say the following: Say, "Bring up the image of the person/situation."

Do 10 to 15 eye movements.

Say, "Notice whatever positive cognition comes to mind."

Say, "Now install the positive cognition _____ (state the positive cognition) with the person/situation's image."

Do 10 to 15 eye movements.

Say, "What do you notice?"

Once the negative affects have been reduced, realistic formulations are much easier to develop. Residual feelings of anger, frustration, regret, or hopelessness have been replaced by clearer thoughts about what can or cannot be done. Positive, creative mulling can proceed without the background feelings of unease, weariness, and ineffectiveness. Daily, weekly, or even career-long burnout can be viewed as the accumulated residual of negative feelings that were not dealt with effectively when they occurred (Daniels, 2009).

Say, "If negativity is not reduced, mentally identify an individual within the EMDR HAP team who could assist you with some EMD, EMDr, or EMDR on this issue."

Say, "Is this a target(s) that you need to take away with you and work on when you get back home?"

Say, *"If so, then mentally identify an individual back at home who may be able to facilitate this."*

Say, *"Be kind to yourself and create an action plan strategy as to how you may be able to get appropriate help and support with this back home."*

Say, *"With these targets you have identified, imagine placing them in a secure container and reinforce this aspect of 'containment' through the use of any slow BLS or the Butterfly Hug to reinforce this."*

Say, *"Consider sharing this with a member of the EMDR HAP team to strengthen your connection with another member of the EMDR HAP team"*

Fifth Stage: Grounding Exercise—Group Share

Say, *"Going around the group, would each of you be willing to share with the group anything from the first three stages that we have just completed such as your contribution to the team, your contribution to an individual, and/or what you have learned about yourself during your EMDR HAP training? It is also fine if you choose to not share your insights now."*

4. Follow Up

The person in charge of psychological well-being identified in Stage 1 as the Group Facilitator is responsible for follow up for each of the EMDR HAP training team members for a minimum three-month period post training. This could either be via telephone, Skype, e-mail, in person, and so on.

Final Comments

As President of EMDR HAP Europe, I receive many requests from members of the EMDR community who wish to become involved in humanitarian assistance programs. Within our EMDR international network, there is an abundance of willing people with big hearts and generous aspirations. In addition, the international demand for EMDR training as part of humanitarian assistance work has never been greater and demand massively outstrips supply. Presently there are EMDR HAP projects throughout Asia, Africa, Europe, North America, South America, and Oceania. No matter how many EMDR HAP trainings there are, there is still not, and probably never will be, enough. To date, several hundred EMDR clinicians have given their time, effort, and energy in the course of bringing EMDR to communities for the purpose of alleviating suffering throughout the world. EMDR cannot develop sufficiently on the international stage without this gift of volunteerism; as such, this gift is the very heart of every EMDR humanitarian assistance program. And yet, as an EMDR HAP and EMDR HAP Europe community, we do have a duty of care to those people who freely give their time to be part of EMDR humanitarian assistance programs. This duty of care requires vigilance and attention toward vicarious trauma. Any trauma work has the potential to disrupt a person's physical, psychological, and spiritual well-being. However, there is also the potential for much internal reward, satisfaction, and personal, psychological, and spiritual positive growth. To return to the words of my therapist "We know what it is, and it is sortable."

Psychometric Measures for Vicarious Trauma

- Derogatis (1983) Symptom Checklist-90 [Revised SCL-90-R]
- Derogatis (1993) Brief Symptom Inventory
- Elliott and Briere (1992) Trauma Symptom Checklist-40
- Figley (1995a) Compassion Fatigue Self-Test
- Foa, Riggs, Dancu, and Rothbaum (1993) Self-Report Post-Traumatic Stress Disorder Scale [PSS-SR]
- Weiss and Marmar (1997) Impact of Event Scale Revised [IES-R]
- Maslach, Jackson, and Leiter (1996) Maslach Burnout Inventory
- Motta, Hafeez, and Sciancalepore (2001) Secondary Trauma Questionnaire
- Pearlman (1996a) Traumatic Stress Inventory (TSI-BSL)
- Pearlman (1996b) Traumatic Stress Inventory Life Event Questionnaire (LEQ)
- Stamm (2004) Professional Quality of Life Scale (ProQOL)

Useful Resources

The Concise Manual for the Professional Quality of Life Scale (Stamm, 2004, 2010) proqol.org/uploads/ProQOL_Concise_2ndEd_12–2010.pdf

Stam, B.H (2010). The Concise ProQol Manual, 2ndEd. Docataile, ID: ProQoL.org Maslach. C, Jackson, S.E, Leite, M.P (1996) Maslach Burnout Inventory Manual (3rd ed.),

Palo Alto, CA: Consulting Phychologistics Press, Inc.

SUMMARY SHEET: Vicarious Trauma and EMDR

3A

Derek Farrell
SUMMARY SHEET BY MARILYN LUBER

Name: _____ Diagnosis: _____

☑ Check when task is completed, response has changed or to indicate symptoms.

Note: This material is meant as a checklist for your response. Please keep in mind that it is only a reminder of different tasks that may or may not apply to your incident.

Vicarious Trauma

Pearlman & Saakvitne's 5 attributes of vicarious trauma: ☐ Completed

☐ 1. Alterations in self-identity and perception
    Description: _____

☐ 2. Alterations in a person's sense of spirituality
    Description: _____

☐ 3. Alterations in personal beliefs and assumptions
    Description: _____

☐ 4. Physical and psychological symptoms
    Description: _____

☐ 5. Impact upon interpersonal relationships
    Description: _____

Symptoms of Vicarious Trauma ☐ Completed

☐ 1. Symptoms of posttraumatic stress disorder: nightmares, sleeplessness, intrusions, avoidance behavior, irritability
☐ 2. Denial of client's trauma
☐ 3. Over-identification with client
☐ 4. No time and energy for oneself
☐ 5. Feelings of great vulnerability
☐ 6. Insignificant daily events are experienced as threatening
☐ 7. Feelings of alienation

☐ 8. Social withdrawal
☐ 9. Disconnection from loved ones
☐ 10. Loss of confidence that good is still possible in the world
☐ 11. Generalized despair and hopelessness
☐ 12. Loss of feeling secure
☐ 13. Increased sensitivity to violence
☐ 14. Cynicism
☐ 15. Feeling disillusioned by humanity
☐ 16. Disrupted frame of reference
☐ 17. Changes in identity, world-view, spirituality
☐ 18. Diminished self-capacities
☐ 19. Impaired ego resources
☐ 20. Alterations in sensory experiences

Are you experiencing vicarious trauma? ☐ Yes ☐ No

If so, what is your vicarious trauma? _____
_____

EMDR Narratives and Vicarious Trauma

The Eight Multiple Narratives within Vicarious Trauma

What are the Multiple Narratives within Your Vicarious Trauma? ☐ Completed

☐ *Narrative 1 – The Narrative of the Story Itself*
_____
_____

☐ *Narrative 2—The Narrator-Who is Telling the Story*
_____
_____

☐ *Narrative 3—The Narration-How the Story is Being Told in Terms of Affect*
_____
_____

☐ *Narrative 4—The Narrative Medium—What Methods are Used to Relate the Narration*
_____
_____

☐ *Narrative 5—Co-narratives—Narratives From the Perspectives of Significant Others*
_____
_____

☐ *Narrative 6—Parallel Narratives—What Other Narratives are Going on Concurrently*
_____
_____

☐ *Narrative 7—The Narrative "Here and Now" or "Time and Place"—Why is this Story Being Told at this Particular Point in Time and Place?*

_____
_____

☐ *Narrative 8—The Narrative Transaction—How the Narrative is Heard by the Listener from the View of the Recipient*

_____
_____

Action Points to Consider in Relation to Addressing Vicarious Trauma ☐ Completed

☐ 1. Either obtain, or utilize existing, good quality, and effective clinical supervision and/or EMDR psychotherapy being clear of the distinction and rationale for both
Notes: _____
_____

☐ 2. Be honest with yourself in acknowledging the difficulties you may be experiencing
Notes: _____
_____

☐ 3. Be open to listening to constructive feedback from clinical supervisors, managers, colleagues, friends, family, and loved ones
Notes: _____
_____

☐ 4. Perform the simple things well in taking care of yourself, maintaining a healthy diet, regular exercise, and generally making time for yourself
Notes: _____
_____

☐ 5. Undertake a complete review of your current client caseload, clinical supervision/ consultation commitments, teaching and learning workload, extra curricula activity, etc
Notes: _____
_____

☐ 6. Revisit 'old comforts'—re-reading your favorite book, watching your favorite films or television series, listening to your music back catalogue of material you haven't heard for a while.
Notes: _____
_____

☐ 7. Give some critical consideration to issues such as work/life balance, areas of 'real' priority in life
Notes: _____
_____

☐ 8. Practice what you preach - Keep a reflective journal, the benefits of which are not just for our clients well-being
Notes: _____
_____

☐ 9. Find physical places and people you can spend some 'quality time' with - make it happen
Notes: _____
_____

☐ 10. Re-introduce yourself and reconnect with social networks and friends
   Notes: _____
   _____

☐ 11. Practice saying 'No' and then feeling 'OK' about it
   Notes: _____
   _____

☐ 12. Give yourself permission to allow somebody else to take care of you just for a while
   Notes: _____
   _____

Root and Branch Review of Personal, Professional, and Spiritual Life ☐ Completed

☐ Personal

Issues: _____
_____
_____

Internal Resources: _____
_____
_____

External Resources: _____
_____
_____

☐ Professional:

Issues: _____
_____
_____

Internal Resources: _____
_____
_____

External Resources: _____
_____
_____

☐ Spiritual Life

Issues: _____
_____
_____

Internal Resources: _____
_____
_____

External Resources: _____
_____
_____

Multiple Narratives and the EMDR Targeting Sequence Plan

Targeting Treatment Plan ☐ Completed

☐ *Target/Vicarious Trauma* _____
_____
_____

☐ *Disturbing Past Experiences* ☐ Age
_____
_____
_____
_____
_____

☐ *Present Triggers*
_____
_____
_____
_____

☐ *Future Outcomes*
_____
_____

☐ *Resources*
_____
_____
_____

☐ *Choose:* ☐ Touchstone Memory ☐ Worst Memory ☐ Other Memory

If dominant symptom is a Negative Belief:

☐ Possible NC: _____
☐ Desired PC: _____

Choose One: ☐ Responsibility ☐ Defectiveness Safety ☐ Vulnerability ☐ Power/Control

EMDR Positive "Stay and Go" Group Exercise Scripted Protocol ☐ Completed

1. Support of the Team—Team Support Person _____

2. Team Meeting—Time of Team Meeting _____

3. EMDR Positive "Stay and Go" Group Exercise with entire group

☐ *First Stage—Being Part of the EMDR Training Team*

Floatback to Training. Contribution made to training: _____

_____

PC: _____
Body Experience of PC: _____
Positive Contribution + PC + Body sensation + BLS

Mental Photograph of Resource: _____

Resource to stay or take away: _____ Stay _____ Take away with me
Add BLS

Float-back over entire training. Positive symbol of being part of team: _____

_____

☐ *Second Stage—Acknowledging Your Contribution to One Individual*

Floatback over entire training. Contribution made to one individual part of training

_____

Contribution: _____
PC: _____
Body Experience of PC: _____
Positive Contribution + PC + Body sensation + BLS

Mental Photograph of Resource: _____

Resource to stay or take away: _____ Stay _____ Take away with me
Add BLS

☐ *Third Stage—Valuing Yourself*

Float-back over entire training: What you learned most about self from this training.

_____

Learned about self: _____
PC: _____
Body Experience of PC: _____
Positive Contribution + PC + Body sensation + BLS
Mental Photograph of Resource: _____

Resource to stay or take away: _____ Stay _____ Take away with me
Add BLS

Summary Sheet: Vicarious Trauma and EMDR

☐ *Fourth Stage: Focusing Upon Your Needs as an Individual*

Float-back over entire training. What negatives you may be holding about the training:
_____

Negatives about training: _____
Body response:
Consider the following:
Target to stay or take away? _____ Stay _____ Take away with me

If needs to remain here would Daniel's Self-Care for EMDR Practitioners sufficient to handle it?
Image of person/situation + 10-15 sets BLS

PC: _____
PC + person/situation's image + 10-15 BLS

Notice: _____

After negative affects reduced, clearer thoughts follow.

If not, identify member of team to assist with EMD, EMDr/EMDR on issue

Resource Individual:_____

Target to work on at home?   _____Yes _____No

Resource Individual at Home With Whom to Work: _____

Create action play strategy for getting help and support at home. Be kind to self.

Action Plan: _____

Place targets identified in secure container + slow BLS

Container: _____

Share with member of team to strengthen connection.

☐ Fifth Stage: Grounding Exercise–Group Share

In group. Share–if you want- anything from first 3 stages (contribution to team, contribution to individual and/or what you learned about yourself during the training).

_____

4. Follow Up

Group Support Person Follows up: ☐ Completed

Worst Case Scenarios in Recent Trauma Response

Ignacio Jarero and Susana Uribe

Introduction

Going to the scene of a disaster is a great service to those in distress and needing assistance. However, this type of work is not one-sided. The survivors' heart-breaking narratives, the sights, smells, sounds, and feelings that assault the sensorium of the mental health responder can range from uncomfortable to overwhelming. It is with this in mind that we offer the suggestions below that we have found helpful during the many years of our work responding to man-made and natural disasters.

Before Deployment

It is important to prepare yourself before you respond to a disaster. These are the types of concerns to keep in mind:

- *Settle Professional and Domestic Issues:* Leave your home and office without unsettled issues in order to be concentrated 100% when you are onsite. The simple things such as leaving pending payments in order, pets in the care of someone trusted, patient appointments cancelled and rescheduled, and the contact information for family and/or friends in case of need, are factors that let us be in the work place completely.
- *Communicate With Service Organizations:* Contact the appropriate authorities to coordinate both logistics (including measures to ensure your personal safety-as much as possible) and interviews with the institutions' personnel or the group(s) to be attended. It is fundamental to communicate with the organizations being serviced. Personal interviews with the institution managers lead us to know approximately what to expect in the field.
- *Be Familiar With the Local Media:* It is of great importance to gather all the information possible before going out on *any* intervention that implies field work, like being familiar with the news transmitted by local media, including TV, newspaper, internet, and radio, in order to have a wider understanding of the situation.
- *Research:* Research is important. Choose the appropriate instruments for your work and make sure that you have copies of what you will need to use.
  Note: We use the Impact of Event Scale-Revised (IES-R) (Weiss & Marmar, 1997) and the Short Post-Traumatic Disorder (PTSD) Rating Interview (SPRINT) (Connor & Davidson, 2001).

- **Team Preparation:**
  1. *Action Plan*
     a. Have a team meeting to elaborate the strategic action plan.
  2. *Physical and Mental Preparation*
     a. *Rest:* Pay attention to getting enough rest in the days before deployment. Appropriate rest allows us to achieve the necessary energy levels to confront the many "worst case scenario" situations we will encounter. It is very important to maintain attention and concentration at all times, since one is exposed regularly to real danger and environmental threats.
     b. *Light and Balanced Nutrition:* Avoid the use of stimulants like coffee in excess, alcohol, tobacco, etc. This allows you to be focused while onsite. Any physical discomfort can interfere with the efficiency of the work to accomplish. Place special attention on the ingestion of minerals and vitamins that reinforce the immune and central nervous system, such as Vitamin C, Vitamin E, and Vitamins B; however, make sure to check with your doctor so you do not self-medicate.
     c. *Moderate Exercising:* While exercising is always valuable, it is vital to be physically rested before doing a worst-case scenario intervention. Any injury or physical pain distracts from the required attention needed in these scenarios.
  3. *Spiritual Preparation.*
     a. *Rituals:* The types of personal, religious and/or spiritual rituals to steady and ground you are essential to your wellbeing in these types of situations. Activities such as religious rituals, chanting, praying, reading something inspiring, lighting a candle, etc. can be helpful-if not essential.
- **Practical Needed Items:**
  1. *Essential Items:*
     ALWAYS bring the following when you deploy to a worst-case scenario situation:
     a. *Food:* Energy/protein bars.
     b. *Clothing:* Easy to wash, clothing appropriate for the area, and comfortable shoes. *Note:* It is preferable for women to be conservative in their clothing, such as loose clothing, with only discrete—bare minimum-jewelry.
     c. *Personal Care Products:* Soap, toothpaste, toothbrush, towel, sunblock, etc.
     d. *Medical Items:* It is helpful to stock a First Aid Kit with necessary medicines for personal use such as the following:
        i. Antihistamines: for any kind of allergy to the environment or bug bite.
        ii. Antacids: sometimes the accessible food is not compatible with our regular diet.
        iii. Analgesics: in case of muscular pains, tooth pain, headaches, etc.
        iv. Anti-diarrhea Medications: the changes of diet can affect the digestive system.
        v. Antibiotics: bring a broad-spectrum anti-biotic as these are generally hard to find without medical prescription.
        vi. Antipyretic Medication: for reducing fever.
        vii. Anti-inflammatory Medicine: for reduction of inflammation.
        viii. Laxative: to treat occasional constipation and restoring regularity.
        ix. Regular Medication: pack enough of the medication you use regularly to ensure that you have enough in case you have to stay longer than anticipated.
        Note: These medicines should be prescribed with medical supervision. This precaution is highly recommended when there is the threat of an imminent epidemic or infection alert due to the disaster.
- "Grab and Run" Suitcase
  1. Grab and Run Suitcase Items: In anticipation of a deployment, it is helpful to have a Grab and Run small suitcase with the following items:
     a. Passport
     b. Food (protein bars)

  c. Water
  d. Personal Care Products
  e. Flashlight
  f. Batteries
  g. Medical items (for at least 2 days)
2. Uses for Grab and Run Suitcase:
  a. After an earthquake, aftershocks are common. It is recommended that you sleep with light clothes on and with the Grab & Run suitcase and flashlight near to you so that you can evacuate quickly as needed.
  Note: It is helpful to have an evacuation rehearsal exercise.
  b. After any type of disaster, there could be a political crisis and you may need to evacuate at any time of night or day for your own protection. Although you might leave your luggage at the hotel or the shelter, always keep your Grab & Run suitcase with you.

During the Intervention

There is a different set of personal needs that are essential to your wellbeing while in these types of difficult and overwhelming situations. Taking care of oneself is fundamental to taking care of others. If you are not dealing with your own personal issues, it will take your attention away from the people and tasks you came to assist.

- *Spiritual Practice:* It is helpful for you to engage in a spiritual practice, in the morning before beginning the day, as it helps you focus on the required activity so that you do not lose sight of your objective/s.
  Note: By acknowledging something bigger than our own egos such as the Divine, God, a Supreme Being, etc., we set the stage to carry out our mission to alleviate human suffering. We ask God for support and protection as well as the support and protection for those we love. In this way, we let go of our worrying about our loved ones for the day and can focus on our objectives.
- *Nutrition:*
  1. *Food:* It is important to eat three meals every day that include more protein than carbohydrates and two snacks (energy bars or a small balanced snack).
  2. *Water:* Abundant hydration with plain water is very important, as you can be so absorbed in your work that you do not realize that you are thirsty. As a result of this phenomenon, drink water every hour, even if you are not thirsty. Have a self-care monitor who is a team member who you choose to look out for you, especially if you have medical issues. For instance, one of our authors remembers being told during the Haiti response, "Dr. Nacho, drink your water!"
- *Work Plan Review:* Review the Work Plan and change it, if necessary. Fieldwork requires flexibility while engaging in tasks, resulting in a better and more efficient performance.
- *Research:* Review with onsite staff and volunteers how the research will be implemented.
  Note: We administer the IES-R and the SPRING before the interventions and at least 7 days post the intervention and if possible 3 months after the intervention.
- *Exercise:* A small walk and stretching are recommended between patients such as going out of the designated room, taking some fresh air/water and/or a bathroom break, etc. Note: Be careful going outdoors if you are in shelters. See Appendix.
- *Midday Meal:* During meals we DO NOT talk about sessions or work, we engage in only nice thoughts and give our complete attention to the nurturing value of our food. It is important to eat more protein than carbohydrates to ensure our stamina for the work that has to be done.
  Note: This recommendation is part of our self-care as it is important to take care of ourselves to be able to take care of others.

- *Power Naps:* After lunch, ALWAYS take a Power Nap, or rest (i.e., take a walk, meditate, or something else that is relaxing to you), if the situation allows. A brief 30-minute nap helps your digestion, clears your mind, and recharges your energy.
- *Team Debriefing:* It is essential to debrief at the end of every workday. In this way, it is possible to address any doubts that you may have, settle any concerns, and address any problems in the response or among each other. Review the work plan for the next day.
- *Emotional Self-Care:*
    1. *Run the Tape:* Each team member runs a mental movie of the day's activities, while doing the Butterfly Hug, to facilitate the Adaptive Information Processing (AIP) system to process any distressful information through our visual, auditory, olfactory, gustatory, and tactile channels.
    2. *Triage:* At the end of the experience, the team leader asks each team member about their physical and emotional states so the leader can evaluate if anything further needs to be done to support the member/s' wellbeing. It is the team leader's job to inform the rest of the team about his/her physical and emotional state as well.
    3. *Role Changing Ritual:* At the end of work every day, we thank our mental health professional part and allow him/her to rest.
    4. *Focus on the Here and Now:* When we return to the hotel/our lodging, generally, before dinner, we take the time to laugh, walk, distract ourselves with simple things, observe the sunset, contemplate nature, drink tea, etc. This practice allows us to be focused on the here and now, maintaining balance between our doing and our being and the realities of the disaster and our own internal resources.
- *Evening Meal:* Dinners are light, nutritious, and work-free. DO NOT talk about patients, painful or stressful situations or any other difficult events of the day.
- *Before Bed Rituals:* It is helpful when you return to your room, to engage in the following practices:
    1. *The Shower Ritual:* This ritual relaxes us and makes us feel fresh. Using relaxing scents in soaps or body washes such as lavender are recommended.
    2. *Personal Spiritual Practice:* Spiritual practices remind you that you are more than just your body and psyche.

    Note: When we surrender to what is bigger than our own egos by a ritual that allows us to connect with the divine (through meditation, prayer, sacred dancing, or any other meaningful ritual), we are reminded of our place in the universe.

    3. *Avoid TV:* Before sleep, it is helpful to take care by protecting yourself from disturbing programs or news. If you cannot avoid TV, it is preferable to choose a comic, peaceful, and/or meaningful selection.
- *Rest:* This is tiring work and it is important to rest for -at least- 8 hours.

After the Intervention

When you complete your involvement with the intervention, it is important for you to continue to take care of yourself.

- *Time Off:* On your way back home, it is helpful to take -at least- one day off, dedicated to doing nice things for yourself such as working out, dancing, going to the movies, seeing friends and family, listening to music, etc.
- *Emotional Self-Care:* It is important to remember that after being exposed to a recent event response, the adrenaline rush decreases and this can lead to feelings of sadness, depression, and anger. You may feel reluctant to return to your daily life that is not as exciting as being in the field of disaster. This is perfectly normal. With this in mind, it is important that you re-involve yourself in your daily activities gradually. It is important that you engage in practices that help support your endorphin release such as cardio-vascular activities, spiritual practices, etc.

- *Research:* Instrument analysis and the writing of corresponding documents should be done very soon after the intervention, so that no information is omitted after returning to normality.
- *Post Intervention Checkup:* The post-intervention team checkup is very important. Sometimes, disturbing sensations, emotions, and thoughts take place in the days that follow. In this meeting, it is helpful to invite an EMDR-trained mental health colleague who was not part of the intervention to evaluate the members of the team and their well-being. If a member/members are having difficulty, using EMDR protocols for recent trauma is helpful.
- *Later Maladaptive Symptoms:* Despite the profound joy and gratitude you may experience after being part of a team that responded to a disaster intervention, it could happen—especially in a man-made disaster- that your believes and/or assumptions of what life is or should be, may be strongly challenged by what you saw and experienced. You may end up feeling that your efforts were worthless, and that your life has no meaning, etc. This may escalate into an existential crisis. If that occurs, it is helpful to seek the advice of a secular or religious counselor to help you feel heard and seen in your feelings of isolation and despair.
Note: This is different than a traumatic memory caused by the intervention. It is more about what happens when you experience—in a despairing way—the awareness of human nature and its limitations.

Appendix: Protection Measures for Mental Health Responders in Shelters and Communities

While working in the shelters and communities in Mexico and Central and South America, the increase in domestic violence, promiscuity, sexual harassment, and abuse of little girls and young women, and even the rape of both male and female helpers has become widespread.

The Mexican Association for Crisis Therapy has developed these important measures to counteract the behaviors described above:

- *Safety First:*
  1. Always assess the potential risks in shelters or communities where you will work and live in. We pay attention to the place where we will be working and/or living, to ascertain if there is risk of any attack, e.g. war between gangs. We always try to stay at places provided by the government and protected by the military.
  2. Do not travel or stay in shelters or communities alone.
  3. Contact people at the shelters and in the communities who are responsible for providing protection.
  4. If there are no designated people to provide protection, it is important to never put yourself in danger. Your safety is first. Look for places to stay safely, even when it entails moving from one place to another.
- *Travel:*
  1. Always travel and stay in small groups of at least three persons.
  2. Always include both men and women in these groups.
  3. In case you have to travel alone, you should contact a family in the community so that you can be accepted as part of the family and have a place where you can be reached.
- *Sleeping Arrangements:*
  1. If you travel with a group, make sure that you have your own place to stay, such as a tent or ranch.
  2. Sleep all together or in a way that no one can be attacked without the others noticing.
  3. Always go with someone when you venture outside, even when going to the toilet or taking a shower.

Summary

Fieldwork is one of the most gratifying experiences we can have as helpers. Nevertheless, it is a very stressful job. It could lead us to develop secondary traumatic stress:

> "... *professionals working with traumatized clients are vulnerable and at risk of developing trauma symptoms similar to those experienced by their clients. Terms used to describe this phenomenon are 'vicarious traumatization' and 'secondary traumatic stress'" (Buchanan, Anderson, Uhlemann, & Horwitz, 2006).*"

When we work in these types of situations, we may absorb the feelings and suffering of the victims we treat. Secondary traumatic stress has the potential to dissolve, destroy and ruin our careers and our lives. As adults, we are responsible for ourselves so it is of vital importance that we understand that principle, as long as we want to keep doing the job we love.

The ideas presented in this chapter are meant to support helpers to be more effective in their work. They present a clear and easy way to organize, prevent, and inoculate you against some of the eventualities that may take place in a disaster intervention. It is also a humble guide based on our experience presented to you with the aim of offering you the gift of our experience.

SUMMARY SHEET:
Worst Case Scenarios in Recent Trauma Response

Ignacio Jarero and Susana Uribe
SUMMARY SHEET BY MARILYN LUBER

4A

Name: _____ Diagnosis: _____

☑ Check when task is completed, response has changed or to indicate symptoms.

Note: This material is meant as a checklist for your response. Please keep in mind that it is only a reminder of different tasks that may or may not apply to your incident.

Before Deployment Checklist

- Settle Professional and Domestic Issues ☐ Completed
  Action Needed: _____
  _____
  _____
  _____

- Communicate With Service Organizations ☐ Completed
  Action Needed: _____
  _____
  _____
  _____

- Be Familiar With the Local Media ☐ Completed
  Action Needed: _____
  _____
  _____
  _____

- Research ☐ Completed
  Appropriate Instruments: _____
  _____
  _____
  _____

- Team Preparation ☐ Completed
    1. Action Plan
        a. Team Meeting ☐ Completed
        Action Plan: _____
        _____
        _____
        _____

    2. Physical and Mental Preparation ☐ Completed
        ☐ Rest
        ☐ Light and Balanced Nutrition
        ☐ Moderate Exercising
    3. Spiritual Preparation ☐ Completed
        ☐ Rituals
- Practical Needed Items ☐ Completed
    1. Essential Items
        ☐ Food—energy/protein bars
        ☐ Clothing—easy to wash, appropriate, comfort
        ☐ Personal Care Products
        ☐ Medical Items
            ☐ Antihistamines
            ☐ Antacids
            ☐ Analgesics
            ☐ Anti-diarrhea Medications
            ☐ Antibiotics
            ☐ Antipyretic Medication
            ☐ Anti-inflammatory Medicine
            ☐ Laxative
            ☐ Regular Medication
- "Grab and Run" Suitcase ☐ Completed
    1. Grab and Run Suitcase Items
        ☐ Passport
        ☐ Food (protein bars)
        ☐ Water
        ☐ Personal Care Products
        ☐ Flashlight
        ☐ Batteries
        ☐ Medical Items (for at least 2 days)
    2. Uses for Grab and Run Suitcase (keep it close always)
        ☐ Evacuation-disaster
        ☐ Evacuation-political

During the Intervention Checklist

- Spiritual Practice ☐ Completed

- Nutrition ☐ Completed
    ☐ *Food—3 meals, 2 snacks*
    ☐ *Water—every hour*

  - Work Plan Review ☐ Completed
  - Research ☐ Completed
  - Exercise—go out of the designated room ☐ Completed
  - Midday Meal—no work talk ☐ Completed

- Power Naps/rest/relax   ☐ Completed
- Debriefing   ☐ Completed
- Emotional Self-Care   ☐ Completed
    ☐ Run the *Tape + Butterfly Hug*
    ☐ *Triage—are you OK?   The leader?*
    ☐ *Role Changing Ritual-thank mental health part & rest*
    ☐ *Focus on the Here and Now*
- Evening Meal-light, nutritious, work-free   ☐ Completed
- Before Bed Rituals   ☐ Completed
    ☐ *The Shower Ritual-to relax, aromatherapy*
    ☐ *Personal Spiritual Practice-you are more than body & psyche*
    ☐ *Avoid TV-protect from disturbing news/programs*
- Rest—at least 8 hours to rejuvenate

After the Intervention Checklist

☐ Time Off-do nice things for yourself
☐ Emotional Self-Care-re-involve in daily life gradually
☐ Research-do write up and analysis soon after return
☐ Post Intervention Checkup-rule-out vicarious trauma, etc.
☐ Later Maladaptive Symptoms-check in for secular/religious help

Appendix: Protection Measures for Mental Health Responders in Shelters and Communities

1. Safety First   ☐ Completed

☐ *Assess risks in lodging*
☐ *No travel or stay in shelter alone*
☐ *Contact responsible people for shelter*
☐ *Never put yourself in danger*
☐ *Travel and stay in small groups of at least 3*
☐ *Include men and women in groups*
☐ *If alone, make contacts in community*

2. Sleeping Arrangements   ☐ Completed

☐ *Own place to stay*
☐ *Sleep together—others notice if attacked*
☐ *Go with someone when go anywhere-toilet/shower*

These ideas present a clear and easy way to organize, prevent and inoculate you against some of the eventualities that may take place in a disaster intervention. It is also a humble guide based on our experience presented to you with the aim of offering you the gift of our experience.

Appendix A: Worksheets

Past Memory Worksheet Script (Shapiro, 2001, 2006)

Phase 3: Assessment

Incident

Say, *"The memory that we will start with today is_____(select the next incident to be targeted)."*

_____
_____
_____

Say, *"What happens when you think of the_____(state the issue)?"*

_____
_____
_____

Or say, *"When you think of_____(state the issue), what do you get?"*

_____
_____

Picture

Say, *"What picture represents the entire_____(state the issue)?"*

_____
_____

If there are many choices or if the client becomes confused, the clinician assists by asking the following:

Say, *"What picture represents the most traumatic part of_____ (state the issue)?"*

_____
_____
_____

Negative Cognition (NC)

Say, *"What words best go with the picture that express your negative belief about yourself now?"*

_____

_____

Positive Cognition (PC)

Say, *"When you bring up that picture or_____(state the issue), what would you like to believe about yourself now?"*

_____

_____

Validity of Cognition (VoC)

Say, *"When you think of the incident* (or picture) *how true do those words____* (clinician repeats the positive cognition) *feel to you now on a scale of 1 to 7, where 1 feels completely false and 7 feels completely true?"*

1   2   3   4   5   6   7
(completely false)   (completely true)

Emotions

Say, *"When you bring up the picture or_____(state the issue) and those words ____*(clinician states the negative cognition), *what emotion do you feel now?"*

_____

Subjective Units of Disturbance (SUD)

Say, *"On a scale of 0 to 10, where 0 is no disturbance or neutral and 10 is the highest disturbance you can imagine, how disturbing does it feel now?"*

0   1   2   3   4   5   6   7   8   9   10
(no disturbance)   (highest disturbance)

Location of Body Sensation

Say, *"Where do you feel it* (the disturbance) *in your body?"*

_____

Phase 4: Desensitization

To begin, say the following:

Say, *"Now, remember, it is your own brain that is doing the healing and you are the one in control. I will ask you to mentally focus on the target and to follow my fingers* (or any other BLS you are using). *Just let whatever happens, happen, and we will talk at the end of the set. Just tell me what comes up, and don't discard anything as unimportant. Any new information that comes to mind is connected in some way. If you want to stop, just raise your hand."*

Then say, *"Bring up the picture and the words____*(clinician repeats the NC) *and notice where you feel it in your body. Now follow my fingers with your eyes* (or other BLS)."

Phase 5: Installation

Say, *"How does____(repeat the PC) sound?"*

_____

_____

_____

Say, *"Do the words____ (repeat the PC) still fit, or is there another positive statement that feels better?"*

_____

_____

_____

If the client accepts the original positive cognition, the clinician should ask for a VoC rating to see if it has improved:

Say, *"As you think of the incident, how do the words feel, from 1* (completely false) *to 7* (completely true)*?"*

1   2   3   4   5   6   7
(completely false)   (completely true)

Say, *"Think of the event and hold it together with the words____(repeat the PC)."*

Do a long set of bilateral stimulation (BLS) to see if there is more processing to be done.

Phase 6: Body Scan

Say, *"Close your eyes and keep in mind the original memory and the positive cognition. Then bring your attention to the different parts of your body, starting with your head and working downward. Any place you find any tension, tightness, or unusual sensation, tell me."*

_____

_____

_____

Phase 7: Closure

Say, *"Things may come up or they may not. If they do, great. Write it down and it can be a target for next time. You can use a log to write down what triggers images, thoughts or cognitions, emotions, and sensations; you can rate them on our 0 to 10 scale where 0 is no disturbance or neutral and 10 is the worst disturbance. Please write down the positive experiences, too.*

"If you get any new memories, dreams, or situations that disturb you, just take a good snapshot. It isn't necessary to give a lot of detail. Just put down enough to remind you so we can target it next time. The same thing goes for any positive dreams or situations. If negative feelings do come up, try not to make them significant. Remember, it's still just the old stuff. Just write it down for next time. Then use the tape or the Safe Place exercise to let as much of the disturbance go as possible. Even if nothing comes up, make sure to use the tape every day and give me a call if you need to."

Phase 8: Reevaluation

There are four ways to reevaluate our work with clients.

1. Reevaluate Since the Last Session

Reevaluate what has come up in the client's life since the last session.

Say, "*Okay. Let's look at your log. I am interested in what has happened since the last session. What have you noticed since our last session?*"

_____
_____
_____

Say, "*What has changed?*"

_____
_____
_____

If the client has nothing to say or does not say much, say the following:

Say, "*Have you had any dreams or nightmares?*"

_____
_____
_____

Say, "*What about_____(state symptoms you and client have been working on) we have been working on, have you noticed any changes in them? Have they increased or decreased?*"

_____
_____
_____

Say, "*Have you noticed any other changes, new responses, or insights in your images, thoughts, emotions, sensations, and behaviors?*"

_____
_____
_____

Say, "*Have you found new resources?*"

_____
_____
_____

Say, "*Have any situations, events, or other stimuli triggered you?*"

_____
_____
_____

Use the material from your reevaluation to feed back into your case conceptualization and help decide what to do next concerning the larger treatment plan.

2. Reevaluate The Previous Target

Reevaluate the target worked on in the previous session. Has the individual target been resolved? Whether the previous processing session was complete or incomplete, use the following instructions to access the memory and determine the need for further processing.

Say, "Bring up the memory or trigger of_____(state the memory or trigger) that we worked on last session. What image comes up?"

___

Say, "What thoughts about it come up?"

___

Say, "What thoughts about yourself?"

___

Say, "What emotions do you notice?"

___

Say, "What sensations do you notice?"

___

Say, "On a scale of 0 to 10, where 0 is no disturbance or neutral and 10 is the highest disturbance you can imagine, how disturbing does it feel now?"

```
0      1      2      3      4      5      6      7      8      9      10
(no disturbance)                                          (highest disturbance)
```

Evaluate the material to see if there are any indications of dysfunction. Has the primary issue been resolved? Is there ecological validity to the client's resolution of the issue? Is there associated material that has been activated that must be addressed?

If you are observing any resistance to resolving the issue, say the following:

Say, "What would happen if you are successful?"

___

If there are no indications of dysfunction, and SUD is 0, do a set of BLS to be sure that the processing is complete.

Say, "Go with that."

Say, "What do you get now?"

___

Check the positive cognition.

Say, *"When you think of the incident* (or picture) *how true do those words* . (clinician repeats the positive cognition) *feel to you now on a scale of 1 to 7, where 1 feels completely false and 7 feels completely true?"*

1   2   3   4   5   6   7
(completely false)   (completely true)

If the VoC is 7, do a set of BLS to be sure that the processing is complete.

Say, *"Go with that."*

Say, *"What do you get now?"*

_____
_____

If there are any signs of dysfunction such as a new negative perspective(s) or new facets of the event or the SUD is higher than 0, say the following:

Say, *"Okay, now please pay attention to the image, thoughts, and sensations associated with_____(state the memory or trigger) and just go with that."*

_____
_____

Continue with the Standard EMDR Protocol until processing is complete.
If the VoC is less than 7, say the following:

Say, "What is keeping it from being a *7?*"

_____
_____

Note the associated feelings and sensations, and resume processing.

Say, *"Go with that."*

Continue with the Standard EMDR Protocol through the Body Scan until processing is complete.

If a completely new incident or target emerges, say the following:

Say, *"Are there any feeder memories contributing to this problem?"*

_____
_____

Do the Assessment Phase on the appropriate target and fully process it. It is not unusual for another aspect of the memory to emerge that needs to be processed.

If the client claims that nothing or no disturbance is coming up (or he can't remember what was worked on in the previous session), and the therapist thinks that the work is probably still incomplete and that the client is simply not able to access the memory, say the following:

Say, *"When you think of_____*(state the incident that was worked on) *and the image_____*(state the image) *and_____*(state the NC), *what body sensations do you feel now?"*

_____
_____

Say, *"Go with that".*

_____
_____

Continue processing with the Standard EMDR Protocol.

If the client wants to work on a *charged* trigger that came up since the last session instead of the target from the previous session, say the following:

Say, *"Yes, this IS important information. Tell me about what came up for you."*

_____

_____

Then assess the magnitude of the trigger. If it is indeed a severe critical incident, then proceed accordingly, using the Assessment Phase to target the new material and return to the original target when possible.

If it is not, then say the following:

Say, *"Yes this is important, however, it is important that we finish our work on _____(state what you are working on) before moving to another target. It is like what happens when you have too many files open on your computer and it slows down, or finishing the course of antibiotics even if you feel okay* (or any other appropriate metaphor for your client).*"*

Fully reprocess each target through the Body Scan and Reevaluation before moving on to the next in order to ensure optimal results.

3. Reevaluate at Critical Points

At various critical points in treatment (before moving on to the next symptom, theme, goal, etc.), reevaluate what has been effectively targeted and resolved and what still needs to be addressed.

Say, *"Now that we have finished this work, let's reevaluate our work so far. Remember_____(state the work you have done). On a scale of 0 to 10, where 0 is no disturbance or neutral and 10 is the highest disturbance you can imagine, how disturbing does it feel now?"*

0   1   2   3   4   5   6   7   8   9   10
(no disturbance)   (highest disturbance)

If the SUD is higher than 0, evaluate what else needs to be done by continuing to work with the disturbance in the framework of the Standard EMDR Protocol.

Also evaluate whether the client has been able to achieve cognitive, behavioral, and emotional goals in his life.

Say, *"Have you accomplished all of the goals that we had contracted to work on such as____(read the list of agreed upon goals)?"*

_____

_____

_____

If not, evaluate what still needs to be targeted such as feeder memories.

Say, *"Please scan for an earlier memory that incorporates_____(state the negative cognition). What do you get?"*

_____

_____

_____

Use the Standard EMDR Protocol to process any feeder memories.
Check if previously identified clusters of memories remain charged.

Say, *"Are there any memories left concerning_____ (state the cluster of memories previously worked on) ?"*

_____
_____
_____

If so, work on the memory(ies), using the Standard EMDR Protocol. Make sure to incorporate the positive templates for all previously disturbing situations and projected future goals. See the Future Template Worksheet Script.

4. Reevaluate Before Termination

Before termination, reevaluate targets worked on over the course of therapy and goals addressed during treatment.

Say, *"Before we end our treatment, let's reevaluate our work to make sure that all of the targets are resolved and goals are addressed. Are there any PAST targets that remain unresolved for you?"*

_____
_____
_____

Or say, *"These are the past targets with which we worked; do any of them remain unresolved? What about the memories that we listed during our history taking and over the course of treatment?"*

_____
_____
_____

Check with the SUDs for any disturbance.

Say, *"On a scale of 0 to 10, where 0 is no disturbance or neutral and 10 is the highest disturbance you can imagine, how disturbing does it feel now?"*

0   1   2   3   4   5   6   7   8   9   10
(no disturbance)   (highest disturbance)

Check the major negative cognitions to see if there are any unresolved memories still active.

Say, *"These are the main negative cognitions with which we worked. Hold _____ (state one of the cognitions worked with) and scan for any unresolved memories. Does anything surface for you?"*

_____
_____

If there is more unresolved material, check with BLS to see if the charge decreases. If not, use the Standard EMDR Protocol.

Say, *"Now scan chronologically from birth until today to see if there are any other unresolved memories. What do you notice?"*

_____
_____

If there is more unresolved material, check with BLS to see if the charge decreases. If not, use the Standard EMDR Protocol.

Progressions can occur during other events or during the processing of a primary target; use your clinical judgment as to whether it is important to return and reevaluate these memories.

Clusters are related memories that were grouped together during treatment planning and can be scanned to identify any memories that were not involved through generalization of treatment effects.

Say, *"Let's check the_____ (state the cluster) we worked on earlier. When you think about it are there any other memories that were not involved that you are aware of now?"*

_____

_____

If there is more unresolved material, check with BLS to see if the charge decreases. If not, use the Standard EMDR Protocol.

Participants are significant individuals in the client's life who should be targeted if memories or issues regarding them remain disturbing.

Say, *"Let's check if there are any remaining concerns or memories concerning ____(state whoever the client might be concerned about). Is there anything that still is bothering you about____(state the person's name)?"*

_____

_____

If there is more unresolved material, check with BLS to see if the charge decreases. If not, use the Standard EMDR Protocol.

Say, *"Are there any PRESENT or RECENT triggers that remain potent?"*

_____

_____

_____

Say, *"Are there any current conditions, situations, or people that make you want to avoid them, act in ways that are not helpful, or cause you emotional distress?"*

_____

_____

If there is more unresolved material, check with BLS to see if the charge decreases. If not, use the Standard EMDR Protocol.

Say, *"Are there any future goals that have not been addressed and realized?"*

_____

_____

_____

Make sure to use the Future Template for each trigger, new goal(s), new skill(s), issues of memory, or incorporating the client's new sense of himself. See Future Template Worksheet Script in this appendix.

Present Trigger Worksheet Script

Target and reprocess present triggers identified during History Taking, reprocessing, and reevaluation. Steps for working with present triggers are the following.

1. Identify the presenting trigger that is still causing disturbance.
2. Target and activate the presenting trigger using the full Assessment procedures (image, negative cognition, positive cognition, VoC, emotions, SUD, sensations).
3. Follow Phases 3 through 8 with each trigger until it is fully reprocessed (SUD = 0, VoC = 7, clear Body Scan) before moving to the next trigger.

   Note: In some situations a blocking belief may be associated with the present trigger requiring a new Targeting Sequence Plan.

4. Once all present triggers have been reprocessed, proceed to installing Future Templates for each present trigger (e.g., imagining encountering the same situation in the future; see Future Template protocols).

Present Stimuli That Trigger the Disturbing Memory or Reaction

List the situations that elicit the symptom(s). Examples of situations, events, or stimuli that trigger clients could be the following: another trauma, the sound of a car backfiring, or being touched in a certain way.

Say, "*What are the situations, events, or stimuli that trigger your trauma*_____ (state the trauma). *Let's process these situations, events, or stimuli triggers one-by-one.*"

Situations, Events, or Stimuli Trigger List

_____
_____
_____
_____
_____

Target or Memory

Say, "*What situation, event, or stimulus that triggers you would you like to use as a target today?*"

_____
_____

Picture

Say, "*What picture represents the*_____(state the situation, event, or stimulus) *that triggers you?*"

_____
_____

If there are many choices or if the client becomes confused, the clinician assists by asking the following:

Say, *"What picture represents the most traumatic part of the_____(state the situation, event, or stimulus) that triggers you?"*

_____
_____

When a picture is unavailable, the clinician merely invites the client to do the following:

Say, *"Think of the_____(state the situation, event, or stimulus) that triggers you."*

_____
_____

Negative Cognition (NC)

Say, *"What words best go with the picture that express your negative belief about yourself now?"*

_____

Positive Cognition (PC)

Say, *"When you bring up that picture or the_____(state the situation, event, or stimulus) that triggers you, what would you like to believe about yourself now?"*

_____

Validity of Cognition (VoC)

Say, *"When you think of the_____(state the situation, event, stimulus, or picture that triggers), how true do those words____ (clinician repeats the positive cognition) feel to you now on a scale of 1 to 7, where 1 feels completely false and 7 feels completely true?"*

1   2   3   4   5   6   7
(completely false)   (completely true)

Sometimes, it is necessary to explain further.

Say, *"Remember, sometimes we know something with our head, but it feels different in our gut. In this case, what is the gut-level feeling of the truth of _____(clinician state the positive cognition), from 1 (completely false) to 7 (completely true)?"*

1   2   3   4   5   6   7
(completely false)   (completely true)

Emotions

Say, *"When you bring up the picture* (or state the situation, event, or stimulus) *that triggers you and those words____(clinician states the negative cognition), what emotion do you feel now?"*

_____

Subjective Units of Disturbance (SUD)

Say, *"On a scale of 0 to 10, where 0 is no disturbance or neutral and 10 is the highest disturbance you can imagine, how disturbing does it feel now?"*

0   1   2   3   4   5   6   7   8   9   10
(no disturbance)   (highest disturbance)

Location of Body Sensation

Say, *"Where do you feel it* (the disturbance) *in your body?"*

_____

Continue to process the triggers according the Standard EMDR Protocol.

Future Template Worksheet (Shapiro, 2006)

The future template is the third prong in the Standard EMDR Protocol. Work with the future template occurs after the earlier memories and present triggers are adequately resolved and the client is ready to make new choices in the future concerning their issue(s). The purpose of it is to address any residual avoidance, any need for further issues of adaptation, to help with incorporating any new information, and to allow for the actualization of client goals. It is another place, in this comprehensive protocol, to catch any fears, negative beliefs, inappropriate responses, and so forth, to reprocess them and also to make sure that the new feelings and behavior can generalize into the clients' day-to-day lives.

There are two basic future templates:

1. Anticipatory Anxiety
   Anticipatory anxiety needs to be addressed with a full assessment (Phase 3) of the future situation.
2. Skills Building and Imaginal Rehearsal
   These do not need a full assessment of target and can begin directly with "running a movie."

Future Template Script
(Shapiro, 2001, pp. 210–214, 2006, pp. 51–53)

Check the Significant People and Situations of the Presenting Issues for any Type of Distress

It is helpful to check to see if all the material concerning the issue upon which the client has worked is resolved or if there is more material that has escaped detection so far. The Future Template is another place to find if there is more material that needs reprocessing.

Significant People

When the client's work has focused on a significant person, ask the following:

Say, "*Imagine yourself encountering that person in the future*____(suggest a place that the client might see this person). *What do you notice?*"

_____

_____

_____

Watch the client's reaction to see if more work is necessary. If a client describes a negative feeling in connection with this person, check to see if it is reality based.

Say, "*Is*_____(state the person's name) *likely to act*_____(state the client's concern)?"

_____

_____

If the negative feeling is not matching the current reality, say the following:

Say, "*What do you think makes you have negative feelings toward*____(state the person in question)?"

_____

_____

If the client is unsure, use the Float-Back or Affect Scan to see what other earlier material may still be active.

If the negative feelings are appropriate, it is important to reevaluate the clusters of events concerning this person and access and reprocess any remaining maladaptive memories. (See Past Memory Worksheet.)

Significant Situations

It is important to have the client imagine being in significant situations in the future; this is another way of accessing material that may not have been processed.

Say, *"Imagine a videotape or film of how*_____*(state current situation client is working on) and how it would evolve*_____*(state appropriate time frame) in the future. When you have done that let me know what you have noticed."*

_____

_____

If there is no disturbance, reinforce the positive experience.

Say, *"Go with that."*

Do BLS.

Reinforce the PC with the future situation with BLS as it continues the positive associations. For further work in the future, see below.

If there is a disturbance, assess what the client needs: more education, modeling of appropriate behavior, or more past memories for reprocessing.

Say, *"On a scale of 0 to 10, where 0 is no disturbance or neutral and 10 is the highest disturbance you can imagine, how disturbing does it feel now?"*

0	1	2	3	4	5	6	7	8	9	10

(no disturbance)   (highest disturbance)

Anticipatory Anxiety

When the SUD is above 4, or when the Desensitization Phase is not brief, the clinician should look for a present trigger and its associated symptom and develop another Targeting Sequence Plan using the Three-Pronged Protocol. (See worksheets on Past Memories and Present Triggers.)

When there is anticipatory anxiety at a SUD level of no more than 3 to 4 maximum, it is possible to proceed with reprocessing using the future template. The desensitization phase should be quite brief.

Say, *"What happens when you think of*_____*(state the client's anticipatory anxiety or issue)?"*

_____

_____

_____

Or say, *"When you think of*_____*(state the client's anticipatory anxiety or issue), what do you get?"*

_____

_____

Picture

Say, *"What picture represents the entire_____ (state the client's anticipatory anxiety or issue)?"*

_____
_____
_____

If there are many choices or if the client becomes confused, the clinician assists by asking the following:

Say, *"What picture represents the most traumatic part of_____ (state the client's anticipatory anxiety or issue)?"*

_____
_____
_____

Negative Cognition (NC)

Say, *"What words best go with the picture that express your negative belief about yourself now?"*

_____
_____

Positive Cognition (PC)

Say, *"When you bring up that picture or_____ (state the client's anticipatory anxiety or issue), what would you like to believe about yourself now?"*

_____
_____

Validity of Cognition (VoC)

Say, *"When you think of_____(state the client's anticipatory anxiety or issue) or picture, how true do those words____(clinician repeats the positive cognition) feel to you now on a scale of 1 to 7, where 1 feels completely false and 7 feels completely true?"*

   1   2   3   4   5   6   7
(completely false)   (completely true)

Emotions

Say, *"When you bring up the picture or_____(state the client's anticipatory anxiety or issue) and those words____(clinician states the negative cognition), what emotion do you feel now?"*

_____

Subjective Units of Disturbance (SUD)

Say, *"On a scale of 0 to 10, where 0 is no disturbance or neutral and 10 is the highest disturbance you can imagine, how disturbing does it feel now?"*

0   1   2   3   4   5   6   7   8   9   10
(no disturbance)   (highest disturbance)

Location of Body Sensation

Say, "Where do you feel it (the disturbance) in your body?"

_____

Phase 4: Desensitization

To begin, say the following:

Say, "Now remember, it is your own brain that is doing the healing and you are the one in control. I will ask you to mentally focus on the target and to follow my fingers (or any other BLS you are using). Just let whatever happens, happen, and we will talk at the end of the set. Just tell me what comes up, and don't discard anything as unimportant. Any new information that comes to mind is connected in some way. If you want to stop, just raise your hand."

Then say, "Bring up the picture and the words____(clinician repeats the NC) and notice where you feel it in your body. Now, follow my fingers with your eyes (or other BLS)."

Continue with the Desensitization Phase until the SUD = 0 and the VoC = 7.

Phase 5: Installation

Say, "How does____(repeat the PC) sound?"

_____

Say, "Do the words____(repeat the PC) still fit, or is there another positive statement that feels better?"

_____

If the client accepts the original positive cognition, the clinician should ask for a VoC rating to see if it has improved.

Say, "As you think of the incident, how do the words feel, from 1 (completely false) to 7 (completely true)?"

1   2   3   4   5   6   7
(completely false)   (completely true)

Say, "Think of the event and hold it together with the words_____ (repeat the PC)."

Do a long set of BLS to see if there is more processing to be done.

Phase 6: Body Scan

Say, "Close your eyes and keep in mind the original memory and the positive cognition. Then bring your attention to the different parts of your body, starting with your head and working downward. Any place you find any tension, tightness, or unusual sensation, tell me."

_____

_____

Make sure that this anticipatory anxiety is fully processed before returning to the Future Template.

The Future Template for appropriate future interaction is an expansion of the Installation Phase; instead of linking the positive cognition with the past memory or trigger, the PC is linked to the future issues. Once the client's work has been checked and the other known issues in the past and present have been resolved, each client has the choice to do a more formal future template installation. The first option is to work with the situation or issue as an image.

Image as Future Template: Imagining Positive Outcomes

Imagining positive outcomes seems to assist the learning process. In this way, clients learn to enhance optimal behaviors, to connect them with a positive cognition, and to support generalization. The assimilation of this new behavior and thought is supported by the use of bilateral stimulation (BLS) into a positive way to act in the future.

Say, *"I would like you to imagine yourself coping effectively with or in_____ (state the goal) in the future. With the positive belief_____(state the positive belief) and your new sense of_____(state the quality: i.e., strength, clarity, confidence, calm), imagine stepping into this scene. Notice what you see and how you are handling the situation. Notice what you are thinking, feeling, and experiencing in your body."*

_____

_____

_____

Again, here is the opportunity to catch any disturbance that may have been missed.

Say, *"Are there any blocks, anxieties, or fears that arise as you think about this future scene?"*

_____

_____

_____

If yes, say the following:

Say, *"Then focus on these blocks and follow my fingers (or any other BLS)."*

Say, *"What do you get now?"*

_____

_____

_____

If the blocks do not resolve quickly, evaluate if the client needs any new information, resources, or skills to be able to comfortably visualize the future coping scene. Introduce needed information or skills.

Say, *"What would you need to feel confident in handling the situation?"*

_____

_____

Or say, *"What is missing from your handling of this situation?"*

_____

_____

If the block still does not resolve and the client is unable to visualize the future scene with confidence and clarity, use direct questions, the Affect Scan, or the Float-Back Technique to identify old targets related to blocks, anxieties, or fears. Remember, the point of the Three-Prong Protocol is not only to reinforce positive feelings and behavior in the future but again to catch any unresolved material that may be getting in the way of an adaptive resolution of the issue(s). Use the Standard EMDR Protocol to address these targets before proceeding with the template (see Worksheets in this appendix).

If there are no apparent blocks and the client is able to visualize the future scene with confidence and clarity, say the following:

Say, *"Please focus on the image, the positive belief, and the sensations associated with this future scene and follow my fingers* (or any other BLS).*"*

_____

_____

Process and reinforce the positive associations with BLS. Do several sets until the future template is sufficiently strengthened.

Say, *"Go with that."*

_____

Then say, *"Close your eyes and keep in mind the image of the future and the positive cognition. Then bring your attention to the different parts of your body, starting with your head and working downward. Any place you find any tension, tightness, or unusual sensation, tell me."*

_____

If any sensation is reported, do BLS.

Say, *"Go with that."*

If it is a positive or comfortable sensation, do BLS to strengthen the positive feelings.

Say, *"Go with that."*

If a sensation of discomfort is reported, reprocess until the discomfort subsides.

Say, *"Go with that."*

When the discomfort subsides, check the VoC.

Say, *"When you think of the incident* (or picture) *how true do those words_____* (clinician repeats the positive cognition) *feel to you now on a scale of 1 to 7, where 1 feels completely false and 7 feels completely true?"*

1   2   3   4   5   6   7
(completely false)   (completely true)

Continue to use BLS until reaching the VoC = 7 or there is an ecological resolution. When the image as future template is clear and the PC true, move on to the movie as future template.

Movie as Future Template or Imaginal Rehearsing

During this next level of future template, clients are asked to move from imagining this one scene or snapshot to imagining a movie about coping in the future, with a beginning, middle, and end. Encourage clients to imagine themselves coping effectively in the face of specific challenges, triggers, or snafus. Therapists can make some suggestions in order to help inoculate clients with future problems. It is helpful to use this type of future template after clients have received needed education concerning social skills and customs, assertiveness, and any other newly learned skills.

Say, *"This time, I'd like you to close your eyes and play a movie, imagining yourself coping effectively with or in_____ (state where client will be) in the future. With the new positive belief___(state positive belief) and your new sense of___(strength, clarity, confidence, calm), imagine stepping into the future. Imagine yourself coping with ANY challenges that come your way. Make sure that this movie has a beginning, middle, and end. Notice what you are seeing, thinking, feeling, and experiencing in your body. Let me know if you hit any blocks. If you do, just open your eyes and let me know. If you don't hit any blocks, let me know when you have viewed the whole movie."*

_____

_____

If the client hits blocks, address as above with BLS until the disturbance dissipates. Say, *"Go with that."*

If the material does not shift, use interweaves, new skills, information, resources, direct questions, and any other ways to help clients access information that will allow them to move on. If these options are not successful, usually it means that there is earlier material still unprocessed; the Float-Back and Affect Scan are helpful in these cases to access the material that keeps the client stuck.

If clients are able to play the movie from start to finish with a sense of confidence and satisfaction, ask them to play the movie one more time from beginning to end and introduce BLS.

Say, *"Okay, play the movie one more time from beginning to end. Go with that."*

Use BLS.

In a sense, you are installing this movie as a future template.

After clients have fully processed their issue(s), they might want to work on other positive templates for the future in other areas of their lives using the above future templates.

Appendix B: EMDR Worldwide Associations and Other Resources

In the Beginning

The EMDR Institute

Web site: (http://www.emdr.com/)
Contact Person: Robbie Dunton (rdunton@emdr.com)

EMDR Worldwide Associations Contact Information

Africa

Algeria

Contact Person: Mohamed Chakali (chakmed@yahoo.com)

Cameroon
Contact Person: Michelle Depré (emdrcameroun@gmail.com)

Ethiopia
Contact Person: Hiwot Moges (hiwot.moges@gmail.com)
Dorothy Ashman (dorothy.ashman@gmail.com)

Kenya
Association: EMDR Kenya (http://emdrkenya.org)

South Africa
Association: EMDR South Africa/Africa
Contact Person: Reyhana Seedat (rravat@iafrica.com)

Zambia
Contact Person: Sue Gibbons (suegibbonsnow@yahoo.co.uk)
Jack McCarthy (jackmcc5@aol.com)

Asia

EMDR Asia Association: An association of Asian National EMDR Associations (http://www.emdr-asia.org)

Australia
Association: EMDR Association of Australia (http://emdraa.org)

Bangladesh
Contact Person: Shamim Karim (shamim.karim@gmail.com)

Cambodia
Association: EMDR Cambodia Association (http://emdrcambodia.org/)
Contact Person: Bunna Phoeun (bunnasyeng@gmail.com)

China—Mainland
Association: China EMDR (www.emdr.org.cn)
Contact Persons: Jinsong Zhang (zhangjsk@yahoo.com)
Lu Qui-Yun (lvquiyun@263.net)

Hong Kong
Association: The EMDR Association of Hong Kong (http://hkemdr.org)

India
Association: EMDR India (www.emdrindia.org)

Indonesia
Association: EMDR Indonesia (http://www.emdrindonesia.org)

Japan
Association: Japan EMDR Association (http://www.emdr.jp)

Korea
Association: Korean EMDR Association [KEMDRA] (http://emdrkorea.com/fine/)

New Zealand
Association: EMDR New Zealand Association
Contact Person: Astrid Katzur (Astrid.Katzur@emdrnz.org.nz)

Pakistan
Association: EMDR Pakistan (http://emdrpakistan.wordpress.com)

Philippines
Contact Person: Lourdes Medina (lcm50us@yahoo.com)

Singapore
Association: EMDR Singapore (http://www.emdr.sg)

Sri Lanka
Association: Sri Lanka EMDR Association (SEA)
Contact Person: Sr. Janet Nethisinghe (jnethisinghe@yahoo.ca)

Taiwan
Association: Taiwan EMDR Association [TEMDRA] (http://www.temdra.org.tw)

Thailand
Association: EMDR Thailand (http://www.emdrthailand.com)

Vietnam
Contact Person: Dr. Carl Sternberg (pv.carl@gmail.com) Ho Chi Minh City

Europe

EMDR Europe Association: An association of European National EMDR Associations (www.emdr-europe.org)

Austria
Association: EMDR-Netzwerk Osterreich (http://www.emdr-netzwerk.at/)

Belgium
Association: EMDR-Belgium (http://www.emdr-belgium.be)

Denmark
Association: EMDR Danmark (http://www.emdr.dk/)

Finland
Association: Suomen EMDR-Yhdistys (http://www.emdr.fi)

France
Association: Association EMDR France (http://www.emdr-france.org/)

Germany
EMDRIA Deutschland e.V. (http://www.emdria.de)

Greece
Association: EMDR Greece (http://www.emdr.gr/)

Ireland
Association: EMDR UK & Ireland (http://www.emdrassociation.org.uk)

Israel
Association: EMDR-IS (http://www.emdr.org.il)

Italy
Association: EMDR Italie (http://www.emdritalia.it)

Netherlands
Association: Vereniging EMDR Nederland (http://www.emdr.nl)

Norway
Association: EMDR Norge (http://www.emdrnorge.com/)

Poland
Association: PTT EMDR (http://www.emdr.org.pl)

Portugal
Association: EMDR Portugal (http://www.emdrportugal.com)

Serbia
Association: EMDR Serbia (http://www.emdr-se-europe.org)

Slovakia
Contact: Daniel Ralaus (ralaus@hotmail.com)

Spain
Association: Associatión: EMDR-España (www.emdr-es.org)

Sweden
Association: EMDR Sverige (http://www.emdr.se/)

Switzerland
Association: EMDR Schweiz-Suisse-Svizzera-Switzerland (http://www.emdr-schweiz.ch)

Turkey
Association: EMDR Derneği (http://www.emdr-tr.org)

United Kingdom and Ireland
Association: EMDR UK & Ireland (http://www.emdrassociation.org.uk)

EMDR Iberoamérica
EMDR Iberoamérica: An association of South and Central America National EMDR Associations (www.emdriberoamerica.org)

Argentina
Association: EMDR Iberoamérica Argentina (http://www.emdribargentina.org)

Brazil
Association: EMDR Brasil (http://www.emdr.org.br)

Chile
Association: EMDR Chile (http://www.emdrchile.cl)

Colombia
Association: EMDR-IBA Colombia (http://emdrcolombia.com)

Costa Rica
Association: EMDR Costa Rica (http://emdrcostarica.wordpess.com)

Cuba
Contact: Alexis Lorenzo Ruiz (alexis.lorenzo@psico.uh.cu)

Ecuador
Association: EMDR Iberoamérica Ecuador (http://emdrecuador.org)

Guatemala
Association: EMDR Guatemala (http://emdrguatemala.org)
Contact: Ligia Barascout (ligiabps@yahoo.com)

Haiti
Contact: Myrtho Marra Chilosi (emdrhaiti2011@yahoo.fr)

Mexico
Association: EMDR Mexico (http://www.emdrmexico.org)

Panama
Association: EMDR Panama (http://emdribapanama.org/)

Puerto Rico
Association: EMDR Iberoamérica Puerto Rico (http://www.emdribappuertorico.org/)

Uruguay
Association: EMDR Uruguay (http://emdruru.guay.org.uy)

Venezuela
Contact: Deglya Camero de Salazar (deglyac@gmail.com)

North America

Canada
Association: EMDR Canada (http://www.emdrcanada.org)

United States
Association: EMDR International Association (http://emdria.org)

Members of EMDRIA Outside the United States

Iraq
Contact Person: Mona Zaghrout (monazag12@yahoo.com; mzaghrout@ejymca.org)

Lebanon
Association: EMDR Lebanon Association
Contact Person: Lina Ibrahin (lina_f_ibrahim@hotmail.com)

Palestine
Contact Person: Mona Zaghrout (monazag12@yahoo.com; mzaghrout@ejymca.org)

Related EMDR Humanitarian Associations

Asia
Japan
Association: JEMDRA-HAP (http://hap.emdr.jp/)

Europe

HAP-Europe
Association: HAP-Europe (http://www.emdr-europe.org)

France
Association: HAP-France (http://www. http://hap-france.blogspot.fr)

Germany
Association: Trauma Aid (http://www.trauma-aid.org)

Spain
Association: HAP-España (http://www.emdr-es.org)

Switzerland
Association: HAP-Schweiz-Suisse-Svizzera-Switzerland (http://www.emdrschweiz.ch)

Turkey
Association: EMDR-HAP Turkey (www.emdr-tr.com)
Contact Person: Senel Karaman (senelkaraman@gmail.com)

United Kingdom and Ireland
Association: HAP UK & Ireland (www.hapuk.org)

Ibero-America

Argentina
Association: EMDR-Programa de Programa de Ayuda Humanitaria–Argentina
Email: emdrasistenciahumanitaria@fibertel.com.ar(Web site under construction at same address)

Iberoamerica
EMDR Iberoamerica (http://emdriberoamerica.org/progamaayudahumanitaria.html/)

Mexico
Asociacion Mexicana para Ayuda Mental en Crisis A.C. (http://www.amamecrisis.com.mx)

North America

United States
EMDR Humanitarian Assistance Program [EMDR-HAP] (http://www.emdrhap.org)

The Francine Shapiro Library

Francine Shapiro Library's EMDR Bibliography (http://library.nku.edu/)

EMDR Journals and E-Journals

The Journal of EMDR Practice and Research—The official publication of the EMDR International Association (http://www.springerpub.com/emdr)
EMDR-IS Electronic Journal (http://www.emdr.org.il)

Related EMDR Information

EMDR Network (http://www.emdrnetwork.org)
EMDR Research Foundation (http://www.emdrresearch.org)

Related Traumatology Information

American Red Cross (www.redcross.org)
The Australian Trauma Web (http://welcome.to/ptsd)David Baldwin's Trauma Pages (http://www.trauma-pages.com)
Children and War (http://www.childrenandwar.org)
European Federation of Psychologists Associations Task Force on Disaster Psychology [EFPA] (http://www.disaster.efpa.eu)

European Society for Traumatic Stress Studies (http://www.estss.org)
Give an Hour (www.giveanhour.org/)
International Society for the Study of Trauma and Dissociation (http://www.isst-d.org)
The International Critical Incident Stress Foundation (http://www.icisf.org)
National Center for PTSD (http://www.ptsd.va.gov)
National Institute of Mental Health (http://www.nimh.nih.gov/health/topics/post-traumatic-stress-disorder-ptsd/index.shtml)
United States National Center for Posttraumatic Stress Disorder (http://www.ncptsd.va.gov/ncmain/index.jsp)
Wounded Warrior Project (www.woundedwarriorproject.org)

References and Bibliography

Adler-Tapia, A. (2012). *Child psychotherapy: Integrating developmental theory into clinical practice*. New York, NY: Springer Publishing.

Adúriz, M. E., Knopfler, C., & Bluthgen, C. (2009). Helping child flood victims using group EMDR intervention in Argentina: Treatment outcome and gender differences. *International Journal of Stress Management, 16(2)*, 138–153.

Alter-Reid, K., Evans, S., & Schaefer, S. (2010, October). *Therapy for Therapists Project: Impact of intensive EMDR treatment post-Katrina*. Paper presented at the EMDRIA Conference, Minneapolis, MN.

American Psychiatric Association. (2000). *Diagnostic and statistical manual of mental disorders-fourth edition text revision*. Washington, DC: Author.

American Psychiatric Association. (2004a). *Diagnostic and statistical manual for mental disorders. DSM-IV-TR* (4th ed., rev. text). Washington, DC: Author.

American Psychiatric Association. (2004b). *Practice Guideline for the treatment of patients with acute stress disorder and post-traumatic stress disorder*. Arlington, VA: Author.

Anderson, M. B., Brown, D., & Jean, I. (2012). *Time to listen, hearing people on the receiving end of international aid*. Cambridge, MA: CDA Collaborative Learning Projects.

Andrews, B., Brewin, C. R., Philpott, R., & Stewart, L. (2007). Delayed-onset posttraumatic stress disorder: A systematic review of the evidence. *American Journal of Psychiatry, 164(9)*, 1319–1326.

Armstrong, K., O'Callahan, W., Marmar, C. R. (1991). Debriefing Red Cross Disaster Personnel: The multiple stressor debriefing model. *Journal of Traumatic Stress 4*, 581–593.

Artigas, L., & Jarero, I. (2009). The butterfly hug. In M. Luber (Ed.) *Eye movement desensitization and reprocessing (EMDR) scripted protocols: Special populations* (pp. 5–7). New York, NY: Springer.

Artigas, L., Jarero, I., Alcalá, N., & Lopez-Cano, T. (2009). The EMDR integrative group treatment protocol (IGTP). In M. Luber (Ed.) *Eye movement desensitization and reprocessing (EMDR) scripted protocols: Basic and special situations* (pp. 279–288). New York, NY: Springer.

Artigas, L., Jarero, I., Mauer, M., López Cano, T., & Alcalá, N. (2000, September). *EMDR and traumatic stress after natural disasters: Integrative treatment protocol and the butterfly hug*. Poster presented at the EMDRIA Conference, Toronto, ON, Canada.

Artwohl, A. (2002). Perceptual and memory distortions in officer involved shootings. *FBI Law Enforcement Bulletin, 10*, 18–24.

Arvay, M. J., & Uhlemann, M. R. (1996). Counsellor stress in the field of trauma: A preliminary study. *Canadian Journal of Counselling, 30*, 193–121.

Ayalon, O. (1976). *Rescue! An emergency handbook*. Haifa, Israel: University of Haifa Press.

Ayalon, O., Lahad, M., & Cohen, A. (1999). *Community Stress Prevention*. Vol 3,4 1999. The Community Stress Prevention Center, Jerusalem Ministry of Education, Kiryat Shmona, Israel.

Ayalon, O. (2003). The HANDS project: Helpers assisting natural disaster survivors. *Community Stress Prevention Centre, 5*, 127–135.

Bar-Sade, E. (2003a). *Early trauma: Revisited and revised through EMDR, the narrative story and the implementation of attachment theory*. Paper presented at the EMDR European Annual Conference, Rome.

Bar-Sade, E. (2003b). *EMDR and children*. The International Trauma Conference, Jerusalem.

Bar-Sade, E. (2005a). *"Attachment cues" as resources in affect regulation enhancement in children's EMDR Processing*. EMDR European Conference, Stockholm.

Bar-Sade, E. (2005b). EMDR and the challenge of working with children. *EMDR-Israel E-Journal*, www.emdr.org.il (Hebrew).

Bar-Sade, E. (2005c). EMDR with children. *EMDR-Israel E-Journal*, www.emdr.org.il (Hebrew).

Baruch, Y. (2009, January). *Mental health assistance in national emergencies: Initial phase*. Paper presented at the International Conference on Crisis as an Opportunity: Organizational and Professional Responses to Disaster, Ben-Gurion University of the Negev, Beer-Sheva, Israel.

Baum, N. (2010). Shared traumatic reality in communal disasters: Towards a conceptualization. *Psychotherapy Theory, Research, Practice, Training, 47(2)*, 249–259.

Beaton, R. D., & Murphy, S. A. (1995). Working with people in crisis: Research implications. In C. R. Figley (Ed.), *Compassion fatigue: Coping with secondary traumatic stress disorder in those who treat the traumatized* (pp. 51–81). New York, NY: Brunner/Mazel.

Beck, A. T., Ward, C., & Mendelson, M. (1961). Beck Depression Inventory (BDI). *Archives for General Psychiatry, 4(6)*, 561–571.

Beebe, G. W., & Appel, J. W. (1958). Variation in psychological tolerance to ground combat in World War II. Washington, DC: National Academy of Sciences.

Birnbaum, A. (2005a, February). *Group EMDR with children and families in South Thailand post-tsunami*. Invited presentation at Bangkok Children's Hospital, Bangkok, Thailand.

Birnbaum, A. (2005b, February). *Group EMDR with children and families following the tsunami in Thailand*. Invited presentation at the EMDR-Israel Humanitarian Assistance Program Conference, Ra'anana, Israel.

Birnbaum, A. (2006, July). *Group EMDR: Theory and practice.* Invited presentation at the EMDR-Israel Humanitarian Assistance Program Conference, Netanya, Israel.

Birnbaum, A. (2007, February). *Group EMDR in critical incident stress debriefing with IDF casualty notification officers: A pilot study*. Invited presentation at the EMDR-Israel Conference on EMDR in the Second Lebanese War, Netanya, Israel.

Bleich, A., Gelkopf, M., & Solomon, Z. (2003). Exposure to terrorism, stress related mental health symptoms, and coping behaviours among a nationally representative sample in Israel. *JAMA, 290*, 612–620.

Blore, D. C. (2009). Blind to therapist protocol. In M. Luber (Ed.), *Eye movement desensitization and reprocessing (EMDR) scripted protocols: Basics and special situations* (chap. 25). New York, NY: Springer.

Blore, D. C. (1997). Reflections on "A day when the whole world seemed to be darkened" changes. *International Journal of Psychology and Psychotherapy, 15(2)*, 89–95.

Blore, D., Holmshaw, E. M., Swift, A., Standart, S., & Fish, D. M. (2013). The development and uses of the "Blind to Therapist" EMDR Protocol. *Journal Of EMDR Practice and Research, 7*, 2, pp. 95–105.

Boel, J. (1999). The butterfly hug. *EMDRIA Newsletter*, 4(4), 11–13.

Brewin, C. R., Rose, S., Andrews, B., Green, J., Turner, S., & Foa, E. (2002). Brief screening instrument for post-traumatic stress disorder. *British Journal of Psychiatry, 181*, 158–162.

Briere, J., & Scott, C. (2006). *Principles of trauma therapy: A guide to symptoms, evaluation and treatment*. Thousand Oaks, CA: Sage.

Bryant, R. A. (2007). Early intervention for post-traumatic stress disorder. *Early Intervention in Psychiatry, 1*, 19–26.

Bryant, R. A., & Harvey, A. G. (2000). *Acute stress disorder: A handbook of theory, assessment, and treatment.* Washington, DC: American Psychological Association.

Buchanan, M., Anderson, J., Uhlemann, M., & Horwitz, E. (2006, December). Secondary traumatic stress: An investigation of Canadian mental health workers. *Traumatology, 12,* 272–281.

Carlson, E, B., & Putnam, F. W. (1992). *Manual for the dissociative experiences scale.* Lutherville, MD: Sidran Foundation.

Cemalovic, A. (1997). *A saga of Sarajevo children: Coping with life under siege.* Stockholm, Sweden: KTH Hogskoletryckeriet.

Chemtob, C. M., & Dutch, H. (2006). *Bi-national trauma response: Building psychosocial resiliency in Sri Lanka [Evaluation report].* New York, NY: UJA Fed NY.

Chemtob, C. M., Nakashima, J., & Carlson, J. G. (2002). Brief-treatment for elementary school children with disaster-related posttraumatic stress disorder: A field study. *Journal of Clinical Psychology, 58,* 99–112.

Cocco, N., & Sharpe, L. (1993). An auditory variant of eye movement desensitization in a case of childhood post-traumatic stress disorder. *Journal of Behavior Therapy and Experimental Psychiatry, 24,* 373–377.

Connor, K. M., & Davidson, J. R. T. (2001, September). SPRINT: A brief global assessment of post-traumatic stress disorder. *International Clinical Psychopharmacology, 16(5),* 279–284.

Crespo, M., & Gomez, M. M. (2011). *EGEP Evaluación Global del Estrés Postraumático.* Madrid, Spain: TEA Ediciones.

Daniels, N. (2009). Self-care for EMDR practitioners. In M. Luber (Ed.). *Eye movement desensitization and reprocessing (EMDR) Scripted Protocols: Basics and special situations* (pp. 399–400). New York, NY: Springer.

de Roos, C., & van Rood, Y. R. (2009). EMDR in the treatment of medically unexplained symptoms: A systematic review. *Journal of EMDR Practice and Research, 3,* 248–263.

Department of the Army. (2006). *Combat and operational stress control: Field manual No. 4–02.51 (FM 8 51).* Washington, DC: Headquarters, Department of the Army.

Department of Veteran's Affairs & Department of Defense. (2009). *VA/DoD evidence based clinical practice guideline for management of concussion/mild traumatic brain injury.* Washington, DC: The Office of Quality and Performance & Quality Management Directorate, United States Army MEDCOM, VA.

Department of Veteran's Affairs & Department of Defense. (2010). *VA/DoD clinical practice guideline for the management of post-traumatic stress* (Office of Quality and Performance Publication 10Q-CPG/PTSD-10). Washington, DC: Veterans Health Administration, Department of Veterans Affairs and Health Affairs, Department of Defense. Retrieved from www.healthquality.va.gov/ptsd/ptsd_full.pdf

Derogatis, L. R. (1983). *SCL-90-R administration, scoring & procedures manual-II* (pp. 14–15). Towson, MD: Clinical Psychometric Research.

Derogatis, L. R. (1993). *Brief Symptom Inventory: Administration, scoring, and procedures manual.* Minneapolis, MN: National Computer Systems.

Dyregov, A. (1989). Caring for helpers in disaster situations: Psychological debriefings. *Disaster Management, 2,* 25–30.

Elliott, D. M., & Briere, J. (1992). Sexual abuse trauma among professional women: Validating the Trauma Symptom Checklist-40 (TSC-40). *Child Abuse & Neglect, 16(3),* 391–398.

Emanuel, Y. (2006, August). Integrating EMDR and a narrative approach in treatment of complex trauma. *EMDR-Israel E-Journal,* www.emdr.org.il (Hebrew).

Errebo, N., Knipe, J., Forte, K., Karlin, V., & Altayli, B. (2008). EMDR-HAP Training in Sri Lanka following 2004 tsunami. *Journal of EMDR Practice & Research, 2(2),* 124–139.

Escudero, A. (2003). *Healing by thinking. Noesitherapy (Biological basis)* (4th ed.). Impreso en Signo Grafico: Valencia, Espana (web-site: http://dr.escudero.com/comprar.html.)

Etherington, K. (2009). Supervising helpers who work with the trauma of sexual abuse. *British Journal of Guidance and Counselling*, 37(2), 179–194.

Everly, G. S., Boyle, S. & Lating. J. (1999). The effectiveness of psychological debriefing in vicarious trauma: A meta-analysis. *Stress Medicine*, 15, 229–233.

Everly, G. S., Jr., & Mitchell, J. T. (2008). *Integrative crisis intervention and disaster mental health*. Ellicott City, MD: Chevron.

Fernandez, I. (2002, Dicembre). I disturbi post-traumatici da stress, fattori di rischio, aspetti diagnostici e trattamento con l'EMDR [The post-traumatic stress disorder factors of risk, diagnostic aspects and treatment with EMDR]. Rivista Scientifica di Psicologia, Sommario 01, 15–24.

Fernandez, I., Gallinari, E., & Lorenzetti, A. (2004). A school-based intervention for children who witnessed the Pirelli building airplane crash in Milan, Italy. *Journal of Brief Therapy*, 2, 129–136.

Figley, C. R. (Ed.). (1995). *Compassion fatigue: Coping with secondary traumatic stress disorder in those who treat the traumatized*. New York, NY: Bruner/Mazel.

Figley, C. R. (2002). *Treating compassion fatigue*. New York, NY: Brunner-Rutledge.

Figley, C. R., & Kleber, R. J. (1995). Beyond the "victim": Secondary traumatic stress. In R. J. Kleber, C.R. Figley, & B. P. R. Gersons (Eds.), *Beyond trauma: Cultural and societal dynamics* (pp. 75–98). New York, NY: Plenum Press.

Foa, E. B., Cashman, L., Jaycox, L., & Perry, K. (1997). The validation of a self-report measure of posttraumatic stress disorder: The Posttraumatic Diagnostic Scale. *Psychological Assessment*, 9(4), 445–451.

Foa, E. B., & Riggs, D. S. (1994). Posttraumatic stress disorder and rape. In R. S. Pynoos (Ed.), *Posttraumatic stress disorder: A clinical review* (pp. 133–163). Baltimore, MD: Sidran Press.

Foa, E. B., Riggs, D. S., Dancu, C. V., & Rothbaum, B. O. (1993). Reliability and validity of a brief instrument for assessing post-traumatic stress disorder. *Journal of Traumatic Stress*, 6(4), 459–473.

French, D. P., & Sutton, S. (2010). Reactivity of measurement in health psychology: How much of a problem is it? What can be done about it? *British Journal of Health Psychology*, 15(Pt. 3), 453–468.

Galliano, S., Cervera, M., & Parada, E. (2004). *El CIPR Procesamiento y Recuperación tras Incidentes Críticos*. Retrieved from http://hdl.handle.net/10401/2975

Galliano, S., & Lahad, M. (2002). Debriefing reconsidered. *Counseling and Psychotherapy Journal*, 3(2), 20–21.

Gawrych, A. L. (2010). *PTSD in firefighters and secondary trauma in their wives*. Hempstead, NY: Hofstra University.

Gelbach, R., & Davis, K. (2007). Disaster response: EMDR and family systems therapy under communitywide stress. In F. Shapiro, F. W. Kaslow, & L. Maxfield (Eds.), *Handbook of EMDR and family therapy processes* (pp. 387–406). Hoboken, NJ: Wiley.

Gelinas, D. J. (2003). Integrating EMDR into phase-oriented treatment for trauma. *Journal of Trauma and Dissociation*, 4, 91–135.

Gilbar, O., Plivazky, N., & Gil, S. (2010). Counterfactual thinking, coping strategies, and coping resources as predictors of PTSD diagnosed in physically injured victims of terror attacks. *Journal of Loss and Trauma*, 15, 304–324.

Grainger, R. D., Levin, C., Allen-Byrd, L., Doctor, R. M., & Lee, H. (1997). An empirical evaluation of eye movement desensitization and reprocessing (EMDR) with survivors of a natural disaster. *Journal of Traumatic Stress*, 10, 665–671.

Greenwald, R. (1994). Applying eye movement desensitization and reprocessing to the treatment of traumatized children: Five case studies. *Anxiety Disorders Practice Journal*, 1, 83–97.

Greenwald, R. (1998). Eye movement desensitization and reprocessing (EMDR): New hope for children suffering from trauma and loss. *Clinical Child Psychology and Psychiatry*, 3, 279–287.

Greenwald, R., & Rubin, A. (1999). Brief assessment of children's post-traumatic symptoms: Development and preliminary validation of parent and child scales. *Research on Social Work Practice*, 9, 61–75.

Greenwald, R. (1999). *Eye movement desensitization and reprocessing (EMDR) in child and adolescent psychotherapy*. Northvale, NJ: Jason Aronson Press.

Greenwald, R. (2000). A trauma-focused individual therapy approach for adolescents with conduct disorder. *International Journal of Offender Therapy and Comparative Criminology, 44*, 146–163.

Grenough, M. (2012). *Oasis in the overwhelm*. New Haven, CT: Beaver Hill Press.

Grieger, T. A., Cozza, S. J., Ursano, R. J., Hoge, C., Martinez, P. E., Engel, C. C., & Wain, H. J. (2006). Posttraumatic stress disorder and depression in battle-injured soldiers. *American Journal of Psychiatry, 163*(10), 1777–1783.

Grossman, D. (2007). *On combat: The psychology and physiology of deadly conflict in war and in peace* (2nd ed.). Millstadt, Illinois: PPCT Research.

Herman, J. L. (1992). *Trauma and recovery*. New York, NY: Basic Books.

Hernandez, D. (2002). DRC: District resource center defined. *Insights*. Retrieved from http://www.openinc.org/newsletters/Insights_2002Fall.pdf

Holbrook, T. L., Galarneau, M. R., Dye, J. L., Quinn, K., & Dougherty, A. L. (2010). Morphine use after combat injury in Iraq and post-traumatic stress disorder. *New England Journal of Medicine, 362*, 110–117.

Holgersen, K. H., Klöckner, C. A., Boe, H. J., Weisaeth, L., & Holen, A. (2011). Disaster survivors in their third decade: Trajectories of initial stress responses and long term course of mental health. *Journal of Traumatic Stress, 24(3)*, 334–341.

Honig, A., & Roland, J. (1998). Shots fired: Officer involved. *The Police Chief, 65*, 16–19.

Horowitz, M. J. (1979). Psychological response to serious life events. In V. Hamilton & D. M. Warburton (Eds.), *Human stress and cognition* (pp. 235–263). Chichester, England: Wiley.

Horowitz, M. J., Wilner, M., & Alverez, W. (1979). Impact of Events Scale: A measure of subjective stress. *Psychosomatic Medicine, 41*(3), 209–218.

Ironson, G. I., Freund, B., Strauss, J. L., & Williams, J. (2002). A comparison of two treatments for traumatic stress: A pilot study of EMDR and prolonged exposure. *Journal of Clinical Psychology, 58*, 113–128.

Ivar, Pivar (2004). Traumatic grief: Symptomatology and treatment in the Iraq War veteran. In The Department of Veterans' Affairs National Center of PTSD, *Iraq War clinician guide* (2nd ed., pp. 75–78). Department of Veteran's Affairs, National Centre for PTSD.

Jarero, I. (2011). *El Desastre Después del Desastre: ¿Ya pasó lo peor? Revista Iberoamericana de Psicotraumatología y Disociación* (Volumen 1, Número 1). Retrieved from http://revibapst.com/DESASTRE-REVIBA.pdf

Jarero, I., & Artigas, L. (2009). EMDR integrative group treatment protocol. *Journal of EMDR Practice and Research*, 3(4), 287–288.

Jarero, I., Artigas, L., & Hartung, J. (2006). EMDR integrative group treatment protocol: A post-disaster trauma intervention for children and adults. *Traumatology, 12*, 121–129.

Jarero, I., & Artigas, L. (2010). The EMDR integrative group treatment protocol: Application with adults during ongoing geopolitical crisis. *Journal of EMDR Practice and Research*, 4(4), 148–155.

Jarero, I., Artigas, L., & Hartung, J. (2006). EMDR integrative group treatment protocol: A post-disaster trauma intervention for children and adults. *Traumatology, 12*, 121–129.

Jarero, I., Artigas, L., & Luber, M. (2011). The EMDR protocol for recent critical incidents: Application in a disaster mental health continuum of care context. *Journal of EMDR Practice and Research*, 5(3), 82–94.

Jarero, I., Artigas, L., Mauer, M., López Cano, T., & Alcalá, N. (1999, November). *Children's post traumatic stress after natural disasters: Integrative treatment protocol*. Poster presented at the annual meeting of the International Society for Traumatic Stress Studies, Miami, FL.

Jarero, I., Artigas, L., Montero, M. (2008). The EMDR integrative group treatment protocol: Application with child victims of mass disaster. *Journal of EMDR Practice & Research*, 2(2), 97–105.

Jarero, I., & Uribe, S. (2011). The EMDR protocol for recent critical incidents: Brief report of an application in a human massacre situation. *Journal of EMDR Practice and Research*, 5(4), 156–165.

Jarero, I., & Uribe, S. (2012). The EMDR protocol for recent critical incidents: Follow-up report of an application in a human massacre situation. *Journal of EMDR Practice and Research*, 6(2), 50–61.

Jelinek, P., & Burns, R. (2012, January). *Pentagon works on new plan to curb sex assaults*. Retrieved from http://www.huffingtonpost.com/2012/01/ll/marines-urinate-corpses-video-afghanistan_n_1200513.html

Jelinek, P. & Burns, R. (2012, January). Panetta assures Afghans of full probe into video. OnlineAthens (Athens Banner-Herald), (http://onlineathens.com/do/not/override/panel/taxonomy/term/43481/2)

Johnson, K. (1998). *Trauma in the lives of children*. Alameda, CA: Hunter House.

Jones, E., & Wessley, S. (2003). Forward psychiatry in the military: Its origins and effectiveness. *Journal of Traumatic Stress, 16(4)*, 411–419.

Jones, E., & Wessely, S. (2005). *Shell shock to PTSD: Military psychiatry from 1900 to the Gulf War*. New York, NY: Psychology Press.

Jones, R. (1997). Child's reaction to traumatic event scale (CRTES). In J. Wilson & T. Keane (Eds.), *Assessing psychological trauma and PTSD* (pp. 291–348). New York, NY: Guilford Press.

Jones, R. T., Fletcher, K., & Ribbe, D. R. (2004). Child's reaction to traumatic event scale-revised (CRTES-R). In J. Wilson & T. Keane (Eds.), *Assessing psychological trauma and PTSD* (2nd ed., p. 523). New York, NY: Guilford Press.

Kabat-Zinn, J. (2012). *Mindfulness for beginners*. CT: Sounds True.

Kaplan G. (1975). *Support Systems in Times of War, The Individual and the Community in Emergencies*. Hebrew University, Jerusalem (Hebrew)

Klingman, A., & Ayalon, O. (1976). Preparing the education system for emergency. *Israeli Journal of Psychology and Counseling in Education (Chavat Da'at), 15*, 135–148. (Hebrew)

Konuk, E. (2009, June). Mental health response and training program for developing countries: The Turkish model. In G. Zaal (Chair), *Diverse*. Symposium conducted at the annual meeting of the EMDR Europe Association, Amsterdam, the Netherlands.

Konuk, E., Knipe, J., Eke, I., Yuksek, H., Yurtsever, A., & Ostep, S. (2006). The effects of eye movement desensitization and reprocessing (EMDR) therapy on post-traumatic stress disorder in survivors of the 1999 Marmara, Turkey, earthquake. *International Journal of Stress Management, 13(3)*, 291–308. doi:10.1037/1072-5245.13.3.291

Korkmazlar-Oral, U., & Pamuk, S. (2002). Group EMDR with child survivors of the earthquake in Turkey. *Journal of the American Academy of Child and Adolescent Psychiatry, 37*, 47–50.

Korn, D., & Leeds, A. M. (2002). Preliminary evidence of efficacy for EMDR resource development and installation in the stabilization phase of treatment of complex posttraumatic stress disorder. *Journal of Clinical Psychology, 58*, 1465–1487.

Kristal-Andersson, B. (2000). *Psychology of the refugee, the immigrant and their children: Development of a conceptual framework and applications to psychotherapeutic and related support work*. Lund, Sweden: University of Lund Press.

Kutz, I., Dekel, R., Schreiber, S., Resnick, V., Dolberg, O. T., Barkai, G., . . . Bloch, M. (2008, November). *The effect of a single session of EMDR on intrusive distress in acute stress syndromes*. Symposium/panel conducted at the 24th annual meeting of the International Society for Traumatic Stress Studies, Chicago, IL.

L'Abate, L. (2004). *A guide to self-help mental health workbooks for clinicians and researchers*. Binghamton, NY: Haworth.

Lahad, M. (2005, October). *1st report to JDC & UJA Fed NY, on the progress of the Tri National project*. Unpublished manuscript, Community Stress Prevention Center, Kiryat Shmona, Israel.

Lahad, M. (2009). *Lessons learnt from the Tri-National project in Sri Lanka following the 2004 tsunami: Focusing on culturally sensitive issues of mental health and psychosocial support and the management of such a project*. Paper presented at the International Conference on Crisis as an Opportunity: Organizational and Professional Responses to Disaster, Ben-Gurion University of the Negev, Beer-Sheva, Israel.

Lahad, M. (2011). *Lessons learned: What was effective post natural disaster training 5 years after the MT training in Sri Lanka was over (2007) field visit and group interview*. A report submitted to UJA Fed. NY and to ITC.

Lahad, M. (2013). BASIC Ph: The story of coping resources. In M. Lahad, M. Shacham, & O. Ayalon (Eds.), *The "BASIC PH" model of coping and resiliency—Theory, research and cross-cultural application*. London, England: Jessica Kingsley.

Lahad, M., Baruch, Y., Shacham, Y., Niv, S., Rogel, R, Nacasch, N., . . . Leykin, D. (2011). Cultural sensitivity in psychosocial interventions following a disaster: A trinational collaboration in Sri Lanka. In R. Kaufman, R. L. Edwards, J. Mirsky, & A. Avgar (Eds.), *Crisis as an opportunity: Organizational and professional responses to disaster* (pp. 129–154). Lanham, MD: University Press of America.

Lahad, M., & Cohen, A. (1997). *Community stress preventions* (Vols. 1, 2). Kiryat Shmona, Israel: The Community Stress Prevention Center, Jerusalem Ministry of Education.

Lamphear, M. (2010). *Effectiveness of the post critical incident seminar in reducing critical incident stress among law enforcement officers*. Doctoral dissertation, Walden University.

Lande, R. G., Marin, B. A., & Ruzek, J. I. (2004). Substance abuse in the deployment environment. In The Department of Veterans Affairs National Center of PTSD (Eds.), *Iraq War clinician guide* (2nd ed., pp. 79–82). Department of Veterans Affairs, National Center of PTSD. Retrieved from: www.ptsd.va.gov

Lansen, J. (1993). Vicarious traumatization in therapists treating victims of torture and persecution. *Torture*, 3(4), 138–140.

Lansen, J., & Haans, T. (2004). Clinical supervision for trauma therapists. In J. P. Wilson & B. Drozdek (Eds.), *Broken spirits: The treatment of traumatized asylum seekers, refugees, war and torture victims* (pp. 317–354). New York, NY: Brunner-Routledge.

Laub, B. (2001). The healing power of resource connection in the EMDR protocol [Special edition]. *EMDRIA Newsletter*, 21–27.

Laub, B. (2009). Resource connection envelope (RCE) in the EMDR Standard Protocol. In Luber, M. (Ed.), *EMDR Scripted Protocols: Basic and Special Situations* (pp. 93–99). New York, NY: Springer.

Laub, B., & Bar-Sade, E. (2009). The Imma EMDR group protocol. In M. Luber (Ed.), *Eye movement desensitization and reprocessing (EMDR) scripted protocols: Basic and special situations* (p. 292). New York, NY: Springer.

Laub, B., & Weiner, N. (2007). The pyramid model—Dialectical polarity in therapy. *Journal of Transpersonal Psychology*, 39(2), 199–221.

Laub, B., & Weiner, N. (2011). A developmental/integrative perspective of the recent traumatic episode protocol (R-TEP). *Journal of EMDR Practice and Research*, 5(2), 57–72.

Lee, C., Gavriel, H., Drummond, P., Richards, J., & Greenwald, R. (2002). Treatment of PTSD: Stress inoculation training with prolonged exposure compared to EMDR. *Journal of Clinical Psychology, 58*, 1071–1089.

Leeds, A. M. (2009). *A guide to the standard EMDR protocols for clinicians, supervisors, and consultants*. New York, NY: Springer.

Levine, P. (1997). *Waking the tiger: Healing trauma*. Berkeley, CA: North Atlantic Book.

Leykin, D. (2012, September). *Crisis management in schools (CIMS) preliminary results from a controlled study* [Research report]. Unpublished manuscript, Community Stress Prevention Center, Kiryat Shmona, Israel.

Litz, B. T. (Ed.). (2004). *Early intervention for trauma and traumatic loss*. New York, NY: Guilford Press.

Lovett, J. (1999). *Small wonders: Healing childhood trauma with EMDR*. New York, NY: Free Press.

Luber, M. (2001, December). In the spotlight. Roger Solomon. EMDRIA Newsletter, 6, 4, 20–21.

Laub, B. (2009). Resource Connection Envelope (RCE) in the EMDR standard protocol. In M. Luber (Ed.), *EMDR scripted protocols: Basic and special situations* (pp. 93–99). New York: Springer Luber, M. (Ed.) (2009a). *Eye movement desensitization and reprocessing (EMDR) scripted protocols: Basics and special situations.* New York, NY: Springer.

Luber, M. (Ed.). (2009a). *Eye movement desensitization and reprocessing (EMDR): Scripted protocols basics and special situations* (pp. 387–392). New York, NY: Springer.

Luber, M. (Ed.). (2009a). *Eye movement desensitization and reprocessing (EMDR): Scripted protocols basics and special situations* (Section, III, pp. 67–106). New York, NY: Springer.

Luber, M. (Scripted by). (2009a). Recent traumatic events protocol. In M. Luber (Ed.), *Eye movement desensitization and reprocessing (EMDR): Scripted protocols basics and special situations* (pp. 387–392). New York, NY: Springer.

Luber, M., & Shapiro, F. (2009). Interview with Francine Shapiro: Historical overview, present issues, and future directions of EMDR. *Journal of EMDR Practice and Research,* 3(4), 217–231.

Ludwig, A., & Ranson, S. (1947). A statistical follow-up of effectiveness of treatment of combat-induced psychiatric casualties: 1. Returns to full combat duty. *Military Surgeon,* 100, 51–62.

Macy, R., Behart, L., Paulson, R., Delman, J., Schmid, L., & Smith, S. F. (2004). Community-based, acute posttraumatic stress management: A description and evaluation of a psychosocial-intervention continuum. *Harvard Review of Psychiatry,* 12, 217–218.

Maguan, S., Lucenko, B. A., Reger, M. A., Gahm, G. A., Litz, B. T., Seal, K. H., . . . Marmar, C. R. (2010). The impact of reported direct and indirect killing on mental health symptoms in Iraq war veterans. *Journal of Traumatic Stress,* 23(1), 86–90.

Maguen, S., Metzler, T., McCaslin, S., Inslicht, S., Henn-Haase, C., Neylan, T., & Marmar, C. (2009). Routine work environment stress and PTSD symptoms in police officers. *Journal of Nervous & Mental Disease,* 197(10), 754–760.

Manfield, P., & Shapiro, F. (2003). The application of EMDR to the treatment of personality disorders. In J. F. Magnavita (Ed.), *Handbook of personality: Theory and practice.* Hoboken, NJ: Wiley.

Marin, P. (1995). *Freedom & its discontents: Reflection on four decades of American moral experience.* South Royalton, VT: Steerforth Press.

Marmar, C. R., Weiss, D. S., & Metzler, T. J. (1996). The Peritraumatic Dissociative Experiences Questionnaire. In J. P. Wilson & C. R. Marmar (Eds.), *Assessing psychological trauma and posttraumatic stress disorder* (pp. 412–428). New York, NY: Guilford Press.

Maslach, C., Jackson, S. E., & Leiter, M. P. (1996). *Maslach Burnout Inventory manual* (3rd ed.). Palo Alto, CA: Consulting Psychologists Press. Maxfield, L. (2008). EMDR treatment of recent events and community disasters. *Journal of EMDR Practice & Research,* 2(2), 74–78. Maxfield, L. (2009). Twenty years of EMDR. *Journal of EMDR Practice and Research,* 3(4), 211–216.

Maxfield, L., Melnyk, W. T., & Hayman, C. A. G. (2008). A working memory explanation for the effects of eye movements in EMDR. *Journal of EMDR Practice and Research,* 2(4), 247–261.

McCann, I. L., & Pearlman, L. A. (1990). Vicarious traumatization: A contextual model for understanding the effects of trauma on helpers. *Journal of Traumatic Stress,* 3(1), 131–149.

McCullough, L. (2002). Exploring change mechanisms in EMDR applied to "small t-trauma" in short term dynamic psychotherapy: Research questions and speculations. *Journal of Clinical Psychology,* 58, 1465–1487.

McFarlane, A. C. (2010). The long-term costs of traumatic stress: Intertwined physical and psychological consequences. *World Psychiatry,* 9, 3–10.

McNally, V. J., & Solomon, R. M. (1999, February). The FBI's critical incident stress management program. *FBI Law Enforcement Bulletin,* pp. 20–26.

Mehrotra, S. (1996). *EMDR an integrated approach to psychotherapy*. Paper presented at the Bombay Psychological Association Annual Conference, Bombay, India.

Mehrotra, S. (2008, June). *EMDR in India*. Keynote and paper presented at the 9th EMDR European Conference, London.

Mehrotra, S., & Geng, W. (2011, February). EMDR in India. *Journal of Xihua University (Philosophy & Social Sciences)*. doi:CNKI:SUN:CDSF.0.2011-02-000

Meichenbaum, D. (1994). *A clinical handbook/practical therapist manual for assessing and treating adults with post-traumatic stress disorder (PTSD)*. Waterloo, Canada: Institute Press.

Melville, A. (2003, April). Psychosocial Interventions: Evaluation of UNICEF supported projects (1999–2001). UNICEF Indonesia.

Mitchell, J. T. (1983). When disaster strikes . . . The critical incident stress debriefing. *Journal of Emergency Medical Service, 13*(11), 49–52.

Mitchell, J. T., & Everly, G. S. (1996). *Critical incident stress debriefing: An operations manual*. Ellicott City, MD: Chevron.

Mitchell, J. T., & Everly, G. S. (2003). *Critical incident stress management: Group crisis intervention* (3rd ed.). Ellicott City, MD: International Critical Incident Stress Foundation.

Modell, A. H. (1976). "The holding environment" and the therapeutic action of psychoanalysis. *Journal of the American Psychoanalytic Association, 24*, 285–307.

Motta, R. W., Hafeez, S., Sciancalepore, R., & Diaz, A. B. (2001). Discriminant validation of the Modified Secondary Trauma Questionnaire. *Journal of Psychotherapy in Independent Practice, 2*(4), 17–25.

Muñoz, M., Vázquez, J. J., Crespo, M., & Pérez-Santos, E. P. (2004). We were all wounded on March 11th in Madrid: Immediate psychological affects and interventions. *European Psychologist, 9*(4), 278–280.

National Institute for Clinical Excellence. (2005). *Post traumatic stress disorder (PTSD): The management of PTSD in adults and children in primary and secondary care*. London, England: NICE Guidelines.

National Institute for Clinical Excellence. (2005a). *PTSD clinical guidelines*. United Kingdom: NHS.

National Institute for Clinical Excellence. (2005b). *Posttraumatic stress disorder (PTSD): The management of adults and children in primary and secondary care*. United Kingdom: NHS.

National Institute for Health and Care Excellence (2005, March). *Post-traumatic stress disorder (PTSD): The management of PTSD in adults and children in primary and secondary care* (NICE Clinical Guideline 26). London, England: National Institute for Clinical Excellence.

National Institute of Mental Health. (2002). Mental Health and Mass Violence: Evidence-Based Early Psychological Intervention for Victims/Survivors of Mass Violence. A Workshop to Reach Consensus on Best Practices. NIH Publication No. 02-5138, Washington, D.C.: U.S. Government Printing Office.

Nikapota, A. (2006). After the tsunami: A story from Sri Lanka. *International Review of Psychiatry, 18*, 275–279.

Norman, S. B., Stein, M. B., Dimsdale, J. E., & Hoyt, D. B. (2008). Pain in the aftermath of trauma is a risk factor for post-traumatic stress disorder. *Psychology Medicine Journal, 38*, 533–542.

Norris, F. H., Galea, S., Friedman, M. J., & Watson, P. J. (2006). *Methods for disaster mental health research*. New York, NY: Guilford Press.

Nouwen, H. (2010, February). *Nouwen & the Ministry of Presence*. Retrieved from http://missionalchurchnetwork.com/nouwen-the-ministry-of-presence/

Ogden, P., & Minton, K. (2000, January). Sensorimotor psychotherapy: One method for processing traumatic memory. *Traumatology, 4*(3), V1(3), 149–173.

Palm, K. M., Polusny, M. A., & Follette, V. M. (2004). Vicarious traumatization: Potential hazards and interventions for disaster and trauma workers. *Prehospital and Disaster Medicine, 19*(1), 73–78.

Parada, E., & Cervera, M. (Unpublished manuscript, 1997). *Psychological first aid response*. Madrid, Spain: ICAS Spain.

Pearlman, L. A. (1995). Self-care for trauma therapists: Ameliorating vicarious traumatization. In B. H. Stamm (Ed.), *Secondary traumatic stress: Self-care issues for clinicians, researchers, and educators* (pp. 51–64). Lutherville, MD: Sidran Press.

Pearlman, L. A. (1996a). Psychometric review of TSI Belief Scale, Revision L. In B. H. Stamm (Ed.), *Measurement of stress, trauma, and adaptation* (pp. 415–417). Lutherville, MD: Sidran Press.

Pearlman, L. A. (1996b). Psychometric review of TSI Life Event Questionnaire (LEQ). In B. H. Stamm (Ed.), *Measurement of stress, trauma, and adaptation* (pp. 419–430). Lutherville, MD: Sidran Press.

Pearlman, L. A., & Maclan, I. (1995). Vicarious traumatization: An empirical study of the effects of trauma work on trauma therapists. *Professional Psychology: Research and Practice, 26*(6), 558–565.

Pearlmann, L. A., & Saakvitne, K. W. (1995). Trauma and the therapist: Countertransference and vicarious traumatization in psychotherapy with incest survivors. New York, NY: W. W. Norton.

Pellicer, X. (1993). Eye movement desensitization treatment of a child's nightmares: A case report. *Journal of Behavior Therapy and Experimental Psychiatry, 24*, 73–75.

Pennebaker, J. W. (1997). Writing about emotional experiences as a therapeutic process. *Psychological Science, 8*(3), 162–168.

Perkins, B., & Rouanzoin, C. (2002). A critical examination of current views regarding eye movement desensitization and reprocessing (EMDR): Clarifying points of confusion. *Journal of Clinical Psychology, 58*, 77–97.

Puffer, M. K., Greenwald, R., & Elrod, D. E. (1998). A single session EMDR study with twenty traumatized children and adolescents. *Traumatology, 3*(2), Article 6.

Purandare, M., Bhagwagar, H., & Tank, P. (2010, July). *EMDR on children affected by the earthquake*. Paper presented at the 1st EMDR Asia Conference, Bali, Indonesia.

Quinn, G. (2009). Emergency response procedure. In M. Luber (Ed.), *Eye movement and desensitization and reprocessing: Scripted protocols basics and special situations*. New York, NY: Springer.

Radloff, L. S., & Locke, Z. (2000). Center for Epidemiologic Studies Depression Scale (CES-D). In *American Psychiatric Association, task force for the handbook of psychiatric measures* (pp. 523–526). Washington, DC: American Psychiatric Association.

Raphael, B. (1977). Preventive intervention with the recently bereaved. *Archives of General Psychiatry, 34*, 1450–1454.

Reddemann, L. (2009). The inner safe place. In Luber, M. (Ed.), *EMDR Scripted Protocols: Basic and Special Situations* (pp. 71–72). New York, NY: Springer.

Roberts, N. P., Kitchiner, N. J., Kenardy, J., & Bisson, J. I. (2009, March). Systematic review and meta-analysis of multiple-session early interventions following traumatic events. *American Journal of Psychiatry, 166*(3), 293–301. doi: 10.1176/appi.ajp.2008.08040590

Rudolf, J. (2012, January). *Marines appear to urinate on dead Taliban fighters*. Retrieved from http://www.huffingtonpost.com/2012/01/ll/marines-urinate-corpses-video-afghanistan_n_1200513.html

Russell, A., & O'Connor, M. (2002). Interventions for recovery: The use of EMDR with children in a community-based project. *Association for Child Psychiatry and Psychology, Occasional Paper No. 19*, 43–46.

Russell, M. C. (2006). Treating combat-related stress disorders: Multiple case study utilizing eye movement desensitization and reprocessing (EMDR) with battlefield casualties from the Iraqi war. *Military Psychology, 18*, 1–18.

Russell, M. C. (2008b). Treating traumatic amputation-related phantom limb pain: Case study utilizing eye movement desensitization and reprocessing (EMDR) within the armed services. *Clinical Case Studies, 7*, 136–153.

Russell, M. C. (2008c). War-related medically unexplained symptoms, prevalence and treatment: Utilizing EMDR within the armed services. *Journal of EMDR Practice and Research, 2*(2), 212–225.

Russell, M. C. (2012, January 27). *Preventing military misconduct stress behavior* [Blog]. Retrieved from http://www.huffingtonpost.com/mark-c-russell-phd-abpp/ptsd-veterans_b_1228546.html

Russell, M. C., & Figley, C. F. (2013). *An EMDR practitioners guide to treating traumatic stress disorders in military personnel*. New York, NY: Routledge.

Russell, M. C., & Figley, C. F. (2013). *Treating traumatic stress disorders in military personnel: An EMDR practitioners' guide*. New York, NY: Routledge.

Russell, M. C., Lipke, H. E., & Figley, C. R. (2011). EMDR therapy. In B. A. Moore & W. A. Penk (Eds.), *Handbook for the treatment of PTSD in military personnel*. New York, NY: Guilford Press.

Russell, M. C., Silver, S. M., & Rogers, S. (2007). Responding to an identified need: A joint DoD-DVA training program in EMDR for clinicians providing trauma services. *International Journal of Stress Management, 14*(1), 61–71.

Russell, M. C., Silver, S. M., Rogers, S., & Darnell, J. N. (2007, February). Responding to an identified need: A joint Department of Defense/Department of Veterans Affairs training program in eye movement desensitization and reprocessing (EMDR) for clinicians providing trauma services. International Journal of Stress Management, 14(1), 61–71. doi: 10.1037/1072-5245.14.1.61.

Samec, J. (2001). The use of EMDR safe place exercise in group therapy with traumatized adolescent refugees [Special edition]. *The EMDRIA Newsletter*. 32–34

Scheck, M. M., Schaeffer, J. A., & Gillette, C. S. (1998). Brief psychological intervention with traumatized young women: The efficacy of eye movement desensitization and reprocessing. *Journal of Traumatic Stress, 11*, 25–44.

Schwartz, A. C., Bradley, R., Penza, K. M., Sexton, M., Jay, D., Haggard, P. J., . . . Ressler, K. J. (2006). Pain medicine use among patients with posttraumatic stress disorder. *Psychosomatics, 47*, 136–142.

Shacham, Y. (2009, January). Challenges in extending help cross culturally [Unpublished PowerPoint slides]. Paper presented at the International Conference on Crisis as an Opportunity: Organizational and Professional Responses to Disaster, Ben-Gurion University of the Negev, Beersheva, Israel.

Shalev, A. Y., Ankri, Y., Israeli-Shalev, Y., Peleg, T., Adessky, R., & Freedman, S. (2012). Prevention of posttraumatic stress disorder by early treatment: Results from the Jerusalem Trauma Outreach and Prevention study. *Archives for General Psychiatry, 69*(2), 166–176.

Shani, Z. (2006, July). *Group EMDR with school children following a traumatic event*. Invited presentation at EMDR-Israel HAP conference, Netanya, Israel.

Shapiro, F. (2006). *EMDR: New notes on adaptive information processing with case formulation principles, forms, scripts and worksheets*. Watsonville, CA: EMDR Institute.

Shapiro, E. (2009). EMDR treatment of recent trauma events. *Journal of EMDR Practice and Research, 3*(3), 141–151.

Shapiro, E., & Laub, B., (2008a). Early EMDR intervention (EEI): Summary, a theoretical model, and the recent traumatic episode protocol (R-TEP). *Journal of EMDR Practice and Research, 2*(2), 79–96.

Shapiro, E., & Laub, B., (2008b, May). *Unfinished-traumatic episode protocol (U-TEP) A new protocol for early EMDR interventions*. Paper presented at the EMDR Europe Annual Conference, London, England.

Shapiro, E., & Laub, B. (2009). The recent traumatic episode protocol (R-TEP): An integrative protocol for early EMDR intervention (EEI). In M. Luber (Ed.), *Eye movement and desensitization and reprocessing: Scripted protocols basics and special situations* (pp. 251–270). New York, NY: Springer.

Shapiro, F. (1989). Efficacy of eye movement desensitization procedure in the treatment of traumatic memory. *Journal of Traumatic Stress, 2*(2), 199–223.

Shapiro, F. (1989). Eye movement desensitization. A new treatment for posttraumatic stress disorder. *Journal of Behavior Therapy and Experimental Psychiatry, 20*, 211–217.

Shapiro, F. (1991). Eye movement desensitization and reprocessing procedure: From EMD to EMDR: A new treatment model for anxiety and related traumata. *Behavior Therapist, 14*, 133–135.

Shapiro, F. (1995). *Eye movement desensitization and reprocessing: Basic principles, protocols, and procedures* (1st ed.). New York, NY: Guilford Press.

Shapiro, F. (2001). *Eye movement desensitization and reprocessing: basic principles, protocols, and procedures* (2nd ed.). New York, NY: Guilford Press.

Shapiro, F. [scripted by M. Luber].(2009). Recent traumatic events protocol. In Luber, M. (Ed.), *EMDR scripted protocols: Basic and special situations* (pp. 143–154). New York, NY: Springer.

Shapiro, F. (2006). *New notes on adaptive information processing with case formulation principles, forms, scripts, and worksheets.* Watsonville, CA: EMDR Institute.

Silver, S. M., Rogers, S., Knipe, J., & Colelli, G. (2005). EMDR therapy following the 9/11 terrorist attacks: A community-based intervention project in New York City. *International Journal of Stress Management, 12,* 29–42.

Silver, S. M., Rogers, S., & Russell, M. (2008). Eye movement desensitization and reprocessing (EMDR) in the treatment of war veterans. *Journal of Clinical Psychology: In session, 64*(8), 947–957.

Skovholt, T. M. (2001). *The resilient practitioner: Burnout prevention and self-care strategies for counsellors, therapists, teachers, and health professionals.* Boston, MA: Allyn & Bacon.

Soberman, G. B., Greenwald, R., & Rule, D. L. (2002). A controlled study of eye movement desensitization and reprocessing (EMDR) for boys with conduct problems. *Journal of Aggression, Maltreatment, and Trauma, 6,* 217–236.

Solomon, R. (2008). Critical incident interventions. *Journal of EMDR Practice and Research, 2,* 160–165.

Solomon, R. M. (1988, October). Post-shooting trauma, *Police Chief,* pp. 40–44.

Solomon, R. M., & Horn, J. M. (1986). Post-shooting traumatic. In J. Reese & H. Goldstein (Eds.), *Law enforcement* (pp. 383–393). Washington, DC: United States Government Printing Office.

Spielberger, C. D., Gorssuch, R. L., Lushene, P. R., Vagg, P. R., & Jacobs, G. A. (1983). *Manual for the State-Trait Anxiety Inventory.* Palo Alto, CA: Consulting Psychologists Press.

Stamm, B. H. (2010). *The Concise ProQOL manual* (2nd ed.). Pocatello, ID: ProQOL.org

Stewart, K., & Bramson, T. (2000). Incorporating EMDR in residential treatment. *Residential Treatment for Children & Youth, 17,* 83–90.

Strupp, H. H., & Binder, J. L. (1984). *Psychotherapy in a new key: A guide to time-limited dynamic psychotherapy.* New York, NY: Basic Books.

Tank, P. (2011). *A presentation on EMDR.* Delhi, India: ANCIPS, EMDR.

Taylor, R. (2002). Family unification with reactive attachment disorder: A brief treatment. *Contemporary Family Therapy: An International Journal, 24,* 475–481.

Tedeschi, R., & Calhoun, L. (1995). *Trauma and transformation: Growing in the aftermath of suffering.* Thousand Oaks, CA: Sage.

Tedeschi, R., & Calhoun, L. (2004). Posttraumatic growth: Conceptual foundations and evidence, *Psychological Inquiry, 15(l),* 1–18.

Tinker, R. H., & Wilson, S. A. (1999). *Through the eyes of a child: EMDR with children.* New York, NY: W. W. Norton.

Turkish Psychological Association. (1999). *Annual bulletin.* Ankara: Author.

U.S. Department of Veterans Affairs & US Department of Defense. (2004). *VA/DoD clinical practice guideline for the management of post-traumatic stress.* Washington, D.C.

Ullmann, E., & Hilweg, W. (2000). *Infancia y Trauma, separación, abuso y guerra.* Auryn colección. Brand. Madrid. (German Original version, 1997).

Van Peski, C. (2006, January). *CSPC crisis intervention training Colombo, Sri Lanka.* Unpublished manuscript, Community Stress Prevention Center, Kiryat Shmona, Israel.

Van Rooyen, M., & Leaning, J. (2005). After the tsunami: Facing the public health challenges. *New England Journal of Medicine, 352,* 435–438.

Weathers, F., Litz, B., Herman, D., Huska, J., & Keane, T. (1993). *The PTSD Checklist (PCL): Reliability, validity, and diagnostic utility*. Paper presented at the annual meeting of the International Society for Traumatic Stress studies, San Antonio, TX.

Weiss, D. S., & Marmar, C. R. (1996). The Impact of Event Scale—Revised. In J. Wilson & T. M. Keane (Eds.), *Assessing psychological trauma and PTSD* (1st ed., pp. 399–411). New York, NY: Guilford Press.

Wesson, M., & Gould, M. (2009). Intervening early with EMDR on military operations. *Journal of EMDR Practice and Research, 3*(2), 91–97.

White, M., & Epston, D. (1990). *Narrative means to therapeutic ends*. New York: Norton.

Wilson, S., Tinker, R., Hofmann, A., Becker, L., & Marshall, S. (2000). *A field study of EMDR with Kosovar-Albanian refugee children using a group treatment protocol*. Paper presented at the annual meeting of the International Society for the Study of Traumatic Stress, San Antonio, TX.

World Health Organization Quality of Life. (1995). Position paper from the World Health Organization. *Social Science and Medicine, 41* (10), 1403–1409.

Zaghrout-Hodali, M., Alissa, F., & Dodgson, P. (2008). Building resilience and dismantling fear: EMDR group protocol with children in an area of ongoing trauma. *Journal of EMDR Practice and Research, 2, 106*.

Zeidner, M., & Hadar, D. (2012, July). Psychoactualia, secondary traumatization among trauma therapists [Hebrew]. *Quarterly of the Israeli Psychological Association*, 42–52.

Additional Readings

Alayarian, A. (2007). Trauma, resilience and creativity: Examining our therapeutic approach in working with refugees. *European Journal of Psychotherapy, Counselling & Health, 9*(3), 313–324.

Altan Aytun, O., Ozcan, G., Ciftci, A., Konuk, E., Yuksek, H., Karakus, D., . . . Vatan Ozcelik, D. (2010, June). The effects of early EMDR interventions (EMD and R-TEP) on the victims of a terrorist bombing in Istanbul. In *Treatment of children/acute stress*. Symposium conducted at the annual meeting of the EMDR Europe Association, Hamburg, Germany.

American Psychological Association. (2003). The road to resilience. Retrieved from http://www.apa.Org/helpcenter/road-resilience.aspx#

Ayalon, O., Lahad, M., & Cohen, A. (1999). *Community stress prevention* (Vols. 3, 4). Kiryat Shmona, Israel: The Community Stress Prevention Center, Jerusalem Ministry of Education.

Bados, A., Toribio, L., & García-Grau, E. (2008). Traumatic events and tonic immobility. *The Spanish Journal of Psychology, 11*(2), 516–521.

Blore, D., & Holmshaw, M. (2009). EMDR blind to therapist protocol. In M. Luber (Ed.), *Eye movement desensitization and reprocessing (EMDR) scripted protocols: Basic and special situations* (pp. 233–240). New York, NY: Springer.

Bremner, J. D. (2005). *Does stress damage the brain? Understanding trauma-related disorders from a mind-body perspective*. New York, NY: W. W. Norton.

Breslau, N., Chilcoat, H. D., Kessler, R. C., & Davis, G. C. (1999). Previous exposure to trauma and PTSD effects of subsequent trauma: Results from the Detroit area survey of trauma. *American Journal of Psychiatry, 156*(6), 902–907.

Brill, N. Q., & Beebe, G. W. (1952). Psychoneurosis: Military application of a follow-up study. *U.S. Armed Forces Medicine Journal, 3*, 15–33.

Brunet, A., Weiss, D. S., Metzler, T. J., Best, S. R., Neylan, T. C., Rogers, C., . . . Marmar, C. R. (2001). The Peritraumatic Distress Inventory: A proposed measure of PTSD criterion A2. *American Journal of Psychiatry, 158*, 1480–1485.

Brymer, J., Layne, P., Ruzek, S., & Vernberg, W. (2006). *Psychological first aid (PFA)*. Los Angeles, CA: National Child Traumatic Stress Network and National Center for PTSD.

Bui, E., Brunet, A., Allenou, C., Camassel, C., Raynaud, J. P., Claudet, I., . . . Birmes, P. (2010). Peritraumatic reactions and posttraumatic stress symptoms in school-aged children victims of road traffic accident. *General Hospital Psychiatry, 32*, 330–333.

Carlson, J. G., Chemtob, C. M., Rusnack, K., Hedlund, N. L., & Muraoka, M. Y. (1998). Eye movement desensitization and reprocessing for combat-related posttraumatic stress disorder. *Journal of Traumatic Stress, 11*, 3–24.

Carmelo, V., Gonzalo, H., & Perez-Sales, P. (2008). Chronic thought suppression and posttraumatic symptoms: Data from the Madrid March 11, 2004 terrorist attack. *Journal of Anxiety Disorders, 22*, 1326–1336.

Cervera, M. (2006). La técnica EMDR en la práctica Terapéutica. La empresa privada en la intervención psicológica en desastres: ICAS. In R. Ramos (Ed.), *Psicología Aplicada a Crisis, Desastres y Catástrofes*. Melilla, Spain: UNED Centro Asociado.

Cervera, M. (2012). La intervencion en situatciones de crisis en las empresas y los primeros auxilios psicólogos. In L. N. Martin & A. S. Sordo (Eds.), *Tratando Situaciones de Emergencia* (pp. 195–210). Madrid, Spain: Pirámide.

Chossegros, L., Hours, M., Charnay, P., Bernard, M., Fort, E., Boisson, D., . . . Laumon, B. (2011). Predictive factors of chronic post-traumatic stress disorder 6 months after a road accident. *Accident Analysis and Prevention, 43*, 471–477.

Creamer, M., Bell, R., & Failla, S. (2003). Psychometric properties of the Impact of Event Scale-Revised. *Behaviour Research and Therapy, 41*, 1489–1496.

Department of the Army. (2009). *Combat and operational stress control manual for leaders and soldiers: Field Manual No. 6–22-5*. Washington, DC: Headquarters, Department of the Army.

Department of Veteran's Affairs & Department of Defense. (2004). *VA/DoD clinical practice guideline for the management of post-traumatic stress* (Office of Quality and Performance Publication 10Q-CPG/PTSD-04). Washington, DC: Veterans Health Administration, Department of Veterans Affairs and Health Affairs, Department of Defense.

Dyregov, A., & Mitchell, J. (1992). Work with traumatized children; Psychological effects and working strategies. *Journal of Traumatic Stress, 5*(1), 5–17.

Fernández-Liria, A., & Rodríguez-Vega, B. (2002). *Intervención en crisis*. Madrid, Spain: Síntesis.

Figley, C. R., & Nash, W. P. (2007). *Combat stress injury: Theory, research, and management*. New York, NY: Routledge.

Finely, E. P., Baker, M., Pugh, M. J., & Peterson, A. (2010). Intimate partner violence committed by returning veterans with post-traumatic stress disorder. *Journal of Family Violence, 25, 737–743*.

Foa, E. B., Keane, T. M., & Friedman, M. J. (Eds.). (2000). *Effective treatments for PTSD: Practice guidelines from the International Society for Traumatic Stress Studies*. New York, NY: Guilford Press.

Galliano, S. (2002). Debriefing reconsidered. *Counseling and Psychotherapy Journal, 3*(2), 20–21.

Gendlin, E. (2002). *Focusing, proceso y técnica de enfoque corporal*. Bilbao, Spain: Mensajero.

Gentry, J. (1999). *Compassion satisfaction manual* (p. 25). Toronto, Canada: Psych Ink Resources.

Gibson, L. E. (2004). *Acute stress disorder: A brief description*. A National Center for PTSD Fact Sheet (www.ncptsd.org).

Gilbar, O., Plivazky, N., & Gil, S. (2010). Counterfactual thinking, coping strategies, and coping resources as predictors of PTSD diagnosed in physically injured victims of terror attacks. *Journal of Loss and Trauma, 15*, 304–324.

Gordon, R. (2007). Thirty years of trauma work: Clarifying and broadening the consequences of trauma. *Psychotherapy in Australia, 13*(3), 12–19.

Grossman, D. (1996). *On killing: The psychological cost of learning to kill in war and society*. Toronto, ON: Little, Brown.

Guenthner, D. H. (2012). Emergency and crisis management: Critical incident stress management for first responders and business organizations. *Journal of Business Continuing Emergency Plan, 5*(4), 298–315.

Horowitz, M. J. (1976). *Stress response syndromes*. New York, NY: Jason Aronson.

Horowitz, M. J. (1999). Signs and symptoms of posttraumatic stress disorder. In M. J. Horowitz (Ed.), *Essential papers on posttraumatic stress disorder* (pp. 1–17). New York, NY: New York University Press.

Institute of Medicine. (2008). *Gulf War and health: Volume 6. Physiologic, psychologic and psychosocial effects of deployment-related stress*. Washington, DC: National Academies Press.

International Association of Firefighters. (2001). *Guide to developing fire service labor/ employee assistance & critical incident stress management programs*. Retrieved from http://www.iaff.org/hs/LODD_Manual/Resources/IAFF%20Developing%20 Fire%20Service%20Labor-Employee%20Assistance%20and%20CISM%20 Programs.pdf

Kimbrel, S., Meyer, K., Knight, Z., & Gulliver. (2011). A revised measure of occupational stress for firefighters: Psychometric properties and relationship to posttraumatic stress disorder, depression, and substance abuse. *Psychological Services*, 8(4), 294–306.

Knipe, J., Hartung, J., Konuk, E., Colelli, G., Keller, M., & Rogers, S. (2003, September). *EMDR Humanitarian Assistance Programs: Outcome research, models of training, and service delivery in New York, Latin America, Turkey and Indonesia.* Symposium conducted at the annual meeting of the EMDR at the annual meeting of the EMDR Europe Association, Istanbul, Turkey.

Konuk, E. (2002). *The August and November 1999 Turkish earthquakes: An EMDR HAP progress report.* The EMDR Practitioner. Retrieved from http://www.emdrpractitioner.net/

Korn, D. L., Weir, J., & Rozelle, D. (2004). *Looking beyond the data: Clinical lessons learned from an EMDR treatment outcome study.* Paper presented at the EMDR International Association Conference, Montreal, Canada.

Kutz, I., Resnik, V., & Dekel, R. (2008). The effect of single-session modified EMDR on acute stress syndromes. *Journal of EMDR Practice and Research*, 2(3), 190–200.

Lazarus, A. (1989). *The practice of multimodal therapy.* New York, NY: McGraw-Hill.

Leach, J. (2004). Why people "freeze" in an emergency. Temporal and cognitive constraint on survival response. *Aviation, Space, and Environmental Medicine*, 75, 539–542.

Levine, P. (2008). *Healing trauma: A pioneering program for restoring the wisdom of your body.* Berkeley, CA: North Atlantic Books.

Shapiro, F. [scripted by M. Luber]. (2009). Recent traumatic events protocol. In Luber, M. (Ed.), *EMDR scripted protocols: Basic and special situations* (pp. 143–154). New York, NY: Springer.

Marks, I. M. (1987). *Fears, phobias and rituals: Panic, anxiety and their disorders.* Oxford, England: Oxford University Press. (Spanish translation: *Miedos, fobias y rituals 1: Los mecanismos de la ansiedad.* Barcelona: Martínez Roca, 1991.)

Marshall, G. N., Davis, L. M., & Sherbourne, C. D. (2000). *A review of the scientific literature as it pertains to Gulf War illnesses: Volume 4 stress.* Prepared for the Office of the Secretary of Defense. National Defense Research Institute, RAND, Santa Monica, CA.

McNally, R. J., Bryant, R. A., & Ehlers, A. (2003). Does early psychological intervention promote recovery from posttraumatic stress? *Psychological Science in the Public Interest*, 4(2), 45–79.

Meyer, E. C., Zimering, R., Daly, E., Knight, J., Kamholz, B. W., & Gulliver, S. (2012). Predictors of posttraumatic stress disorder and other psychological symptoms in trauma-exposed firefighters. *Psychological Services*, 9(1), 1–15.

Mitchell, J. T., & Everly, G. S. (2001). Critical incident stress management and critical incident stress debriefing: Evolution, effects and outcomes. In B. Raphael & J. Wilson (Eds.), *Psychological debriefing: Theory, practice and evidence.* Cambridge, UK: Cambridge University Press.

Murphy, S. A., Bond, G. E., Beaton, R. D., Murphy, J., & Clark, L. C. (2002). Lifestyle practices and occupational stressors as predictors of health outcomes in urban firefighters. *International Journal of Stress Management*, 9(4), 311–327.

Neria, Y., DiGrande, L., & Adams, B. G. (2011). Posttraumatic stress disorder following the September 11, 2001, terrorist attacks: A review of the literature among highly exposed populations. *American Psychologist*, 66(6), 429–446.

Ogden, P., Minton, K., & Pain, C. (2006). *Trauma and the body: A sensorimotor approach to psychotherapy.* New York, NY: W. W. Norton.

Rothschild, B. (2006). *Help for the helper: Self-care strategies for managing burnout and stress.* New York, NY: W. W. Norton.

Russell, M. C. (2008a). Scientific resistance to research, training, and utilization of EMDR therapy in treating post-war disorders. *Social Science and Medicine*, 67(11), 1737–1746.

Russell, M. C., & Friedberg, F. (2009). Training, treatment access and research on trauma intervention in the armed services. *Journal of EMDR Practice and Research*, 3, 24–31.

Seyle, H., & Fortier, C. (1950). Adaptive reaction to stress. *Psychosomatic Medicine 12(3)*, 149–157.

Shapiro, E. (2007). 4 Elements exercise. *Journal of EMDR Practice and Research*, 2, 113–115.

Shapiro, E. (2012). EMDR and early psychological intervention following trauma. *European Journal of Applied Psychology (ERAP)*, V. 62(4), 241–251.

Shapiro, F. (1993). Eye movement desensitization and reprocessing (EMDR). *Journal of Traumatic Stress*, 6, 417–421.

Shapiro, F. (1999). Eye movement desensitization and reprocessing (EMDR) and the anxiety disorders: Clinical and research implications of an integrated psychotherapy treatment. *Journal of Anxiety Disorders, 13*(1–2, Excerpt), 35–67.

Shapiro, F. (2004). *Military and post-disaster field manual.* Hamden, CT: EMDR Humanitarian Assistance Program.

Shapiro, F. (In press). Protocol for recent traumatic events. In M. Luber (Ed.), *Implementing EMDR early mental health interventions for man-made and natural disasters: Models, scripted protocols and summary sheets.* New York, NY: Springer.

Silver, S., & Rogers, S. (2001). *Light in the heart of darkness: EMDR and the treatment of war and terrorism survivors.* New York, NY: W. W. Norton.

Slonim, D. (2010, July). *Post traumatic stress disorder.* Paper presented at the NATO Science for Peace conference, Istanbul, Turkey.

Sosa, C. D., & Capafons, J. (2005). *Estrés Postraumático.* Madrid, Spain: Síntesis.

Stapert, M., & Verliefde, E. (2008). *Focusing with children. The art of communicating with children at school and at home.* United Kingdom: PCCS Books. (Spanish versión 2011.)

Ullmann, E., & Hilweg, W. (2000). *Infancia y Trauma, separación, abuso y guerra.* Auryn colección. Madrid: Brand. (German Original version, 1997.) Wittman, L., Zehnder, D., Schredl, M., Jenni, O. G., & Landolt, M. A. (2010). Posttraumatic nightmares and psychopathology in children after a road traffic accidents. *Journal of Traumatic Stress*, 23(2), 232–239.

Yehuda, R. (1999). *Risk factors for posttraumatic stress disorder.* Washington, DC: American Psychiatric Association. Yehuda, R. (2001). Biology of post traumatic stress disorder. *Psychiatric Clinics of North America, 62*(Suppl. 17), 41–46.

Zayfer, C., & Becker, C. B. (2007). *Cognitive—Behavioral therapy for PTSD.* New York, NY: Guilford Press. (Spanish versión, 2008. México: El Manual Moderno.)

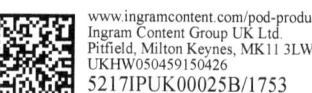

www.ingramcontent.com/pod-product-compliance
Ingram Content Group UK Ltd.
Pitfield, Milton Keynes, MK11 3LW, UK
UKHW050459150426
5217IPUK00025B/1753